Loss and Bereavement in Childbearing

Rosemary Mander
MSc, PhD, RGN, SCM, MTD
Lecturer
Department of Nursing Studies
University of Edinburgh

OXFORD

BLACKWELL SCIENTIFIC PUBLICATIONS

LONDON EDINBURGH BOSTON

MELBOURNE PARIS BERLIN VIENNA

© 1994 by
Blackwell Scientific Publications
Editorial Offices:
Osney Mead, Oxford OX2 0EL
25 John Street, London WC1N 2BL
23 Ainslie Place, Edinburgh EH3 6AJ
238 Main Street, Cambridge,
  Massachusetts 02142, USA
54 University Street, Carlton,
  Victoria 3053, Australia

Other Editorial Offices:
Librairie Arnette SA
1, rue de Lille
75007 Paris
France

Blackwell Wissenschafts-Verlag GmbH
Kurfürstendamm 57
10707 Berlin
Germany

Blackwell MZV
Feldgasse 13
A-1238 Wien
Austria

First published 1994

Set by DP Photosetting, Aylesbury, Bucks
Printed and bound in Great Britain by
Hartnolls Ltd, Bodmin, Cornwall

DISTRIBUTORS

Marston Book Services Ltd
PO Box 87
Oxford OX2 0DT
(*Orders:* Tel: 0865 791155
          Fax: 0865 791927
          Telex: 837515)

USA
  Blackwell Scientific Publications, Inc.
  238 Main Street
  Cambridge, MA 02142
  (*Orders:* Tel: 800 759-6102
             617 876-7000)

Canada
  Times Mirror Professional Publishing, Ltd
  130 Flaska Drive
  Markham, Ontario L6G 1B8
  (*Orders:* Tel: 800 268-4178
             416 470-6739)

Australia
  Blackwell Scientific Publications Pty Ltd
  54 University Street
  Carlton, Victoria 3053
  (*Orders:* Tel: (03) 347-5552)

British Library
Cataloguing in Publication Data

A catalogue record for this book is available
from the British Library

ISBN 0–632–03826–8

Library of Congress
Cataloging in Publication Data
Mander, Rosemary.
    Loss and Bereavement in childbearing/
Rosemary Mander.
       p. cm.
    Includes bibliographical references and
index.
    ISBN 0-632-03826-8
    1. Miscarriage—Psychological aspects.
  2. Stillbirth—Psychological aspects.
  3. Fetal death—Psychological aspects.
  4. Bereavement—Psychological aspects.
  5. Medical personnel and patient.   I. Title.
  RG648.M345   1994
  155.9'37—dc20   94-13658
                                            CIP

Contents

Preface

How do I introduce loss?

I don't think I do.

I don't need to make the introduction because you know loss already. Was it when your grandmother died? Was it when your first child was miscarried? Was it when a mother you'd been caring for had an unexpected stillbirth? Was it when your childish idealisation of your own mother was replaced by your realisation of her humanity? Was it when your first 'steady' told you that they were 'chucking' you? Was it the day you got home to find that a burglar had messed up your bedroom? Was it perhaps when you didn't come top in the exams? Was it when your partner was made redundant?

We all know loss. It is fundamental to life. You might say it is a fact of life. And like so many facts of life, together with the grief which follows, it helps us to grow and to develop into the people we are. Inevitably our minds home-in first of all on the major losses, often of those we love. But as we have seen already there is no shortage of other examples.

It is neither easy nor necessary to separate out our personal losses from those we face in the course of our work as midwives or carers. The painful memories which we may regard as safely out of the way have a nasty habit of reappearing at surprising and discomforting moments. In the course of my work I have certainly found that my own losses, either actual or potential, have been brought into sharper focus by my reading, writing and caring. There has been more than one occasion when I have found tears dropping on to a book or on to my computer keyboard.

Because loss is so crucially personal, I use the first person. I make no apology for this. It serves to remind us that reading and learning is about sharing knowledge and ideas. Thus, the ideas and experience which I offer in this book interact with those of you, the reader. Although I have written this book it is not because I claim unique expertise in this area. I attempt as far as possible to avoid a prescriptive, dogmatic, 'expert' or 'cookbook' approach. Is there a recipe for effective care of a grieving mother? Like those we care for, we all have our own unique expertise. In certain situations, such as her grief, only the mother knows what it is like. Only by accepting how she sees it do we have a basis from which to begin to help her.

While recognising that our care is increasingly orientated towards the care of the family, I emphasise throughout this book our care of the mother. This is because the mother is invariably intimately involved with loss in childbearing, while others may either be less involved or else differently involved. I concentrate on her reactions and difficulties and assume that many of her feelings are shared by those close to her. I mention other family members when they may be affected differently. It is possible that others near her, such as the father, may have similar, or perhaps even more extreme, reactions, but I address his orientation and response in Chapter 6.

This book opens with a chapter examining events around the time of birth. These events may happen when a baby dies and they may happen if the baby is alive and well. I suggest that neither outcome is uniformly negative or positive.

Because of its importance in all aspects of our work, including when there is grief, the chapter on our use and misuse of research is next. In Chapter 3 I consider the ways in which loss in childbearing may manifest itself in order to set the scene for the next chapter on the principles of care. Four chapters on specific aspects of care follow: counselling, other family members, the mother who is HIV-positive, and the care of the family with a baby in the neonatal unit.

In Chapters 9 and 10 we hold up a mirror to look at our own responses to loss. These lead us to think about certain other carers whose input should not be underestimated; these are the lay supporters. Finally, we look forward to the mother's experience in any future pregnancy.

In writing this book I aim to help the midwife caring for a mother experiencing any form of loss in childbearing. I hope, through this book, to prevent the additional suffering which a woman may face when her carers are unable to provide appropriate care. I hope, also, to minimise the feelings which the midwife encounters when she knows that the care being provided is less than it should be. Although we ordinarily perceive bereavement as a totally negative event with unpleasant or unhealthy consequences, this book will help those involved to begin the process of grieving in the most favourable circumstances.

Acknowledgements

I would like to acknowledge the generous financial support provided by the Iolanthe Trust, which enabled me to undertake the study mentioned in this book. I am grateful to the mothers and the midwives who generously gave of their experience and their expertise, their time and their tears.

I also acknowledge the help of Claire Greig and of my colleagues Sarah Baggaley and Nick Watson for their comments on some of the chapters. I particularly appreciate the help of Iain Abbot who not only read chapters but also helped me in other ways too numerous to recall.

List of Abbreviations

A&E	Accident and Emergency department
AID	Artificial Insemination by Donor
AIDS	Acquired Immune Deficiency Syndrome
DIC	Disseminated Intravascular Coagulation
GAS	General Adaptation Syndrome
GP	general practitioner
HIV	Human Immunodeficiency Virus
HV	health visitor
ITU	Intensive Therapy Unit
IUD	intra-uterine death
IVDU	intravenous drug user
LBW	low birth weight
NNICU	neonatal intensive care unit
NNU	neonatal unit
PM	post-mortem
POC	products of conception
PSE	Present State Examination
RECs	research ethics committees
SANDS	Stillbirth and Neonatal Death Society
SCBU	Special Care Baby Unit
SIDS	Sudden Infant Death Syndrome
TAMBA	Twins and Multiple Births Association
TOP	termination of pregnancy

Chapter 1
Grieving, Mourning, Loving and Losing

In this chapter I consider the meaning of loss and begin to apply loss to childbearing. I think, first, about the words which we use and then move on to look at the healthy and unhealthy ways in which grief may progress. Next, I think about love, which is the essential precursor to grief, and how loving relationships begin. These thoughts lead into consideration of the feelings of loss which may feature in happy, successful childbearing.

Our attitude to death has changed over the past hundred years. In current western society our attitude to loss through death tends to be similar to the Victorian attitude to sex – the ultimate unmentionable (Sheard, 1984). It may be that our attitudes to these two essential aspects of human life have become reversed. This is partly because our society now tends to focus more on young, healthy, sexually active people, despite our increasing proportion of elderly people. Because of this altered focus and the changing pattern of health and illness, the spectre of death is no longer our constant companion. The result is that the taboos have become transposed (Gorer, 1965).

Despite these changing attitudes the fact remains that death is an essential part of life. Our grief over the loss of a loved one is the price that we must pay for the pleasure which that love brought with it; 'we cannot fully know the rich textured experience of being alive until we learn to look calmly into the face of death' (Campbell, 1979). The reality and proximity of loss is demonstrated when Campbell shows us how, in order to grow and develop into mature human beings, we must progress through certain phases involving the loss of aspects of our earlier selves. He evidences the loss of our childhood selves, our fantasy parents, our youthful expectations and the world as we have come to know it. Each loss needs to be mourned in order to recognise its passage and prepare for the move on to the next phase in our lives.

The inevitability of death still tends to be avoided if not ignored, although the topic is beginning to be opened up by researchers and other writers. It may be that, as the population becomes older, death in old age is becoming a more widely-recognised and accepted event.

1

Whether this acceptance applies to death and loss at the opposite extreme of age is less certain.

Words and meanings

Our understanding of the experience of the person who has been bereaved has grown vastly during the past four decades. This growth has been due largely to the interest of researchers and other workers from a wide range of disciplines, including psychology, physiology, psychiatry and sociology, as well as nursing and midwifery. The result of such a heterogeneous input into our knowledge-base is not only a more comprehensive picture of this experience, but also greater diversity in the meanings of the basic terms we use about loss and bereavement.

For this reason I begin by explaining the meanings of these terms as I use them.

Grief

Although it may have many social, financial and practical as well as other implications, the essence of the experience of loss lies in the person's psychological or emotional response (Rando, 1986). This is what we call grief. It is quite specific and is intensely personal and individual. These aspects must not be allowed to distract our attention from both the complexity of this emotion and the depth of the person's feelings. Osterweis *et al.* (1984) broaden the scope of grief marginally by including in it those behaviours which are directly associated; in this way weeping may be regarded as a crucial part of grief.

Grieving

The changes or developments in the person's emotional state are known as grieving or the grieving process. The factors affecting how grief develops have come to underpin our knowledge of this area, as I show later in this chapter.

Mourning

Whereas grief and grieving focus solely and narrowly on the person's emotional state, mourning involves the wide-ranging, more socially-orientated manifestations of loss. It is through mourning that we are able to undo the psychological bonds that have cemented our relationships with those who have died. Many of the rituals or rites of passage associated with loss are culturally determined, varying according to ethnic origin, socioeconomic class, prevailing social attitudes and religious persuasion. Mourning provides an opportunity for the expression of respect for the one who is lost. It also shows the sorrow of the community and support for those most intimately affected by the loss.

Clark (1991) states that mourning serves to confirm the relationships between those who remain and strengthen the continuing ties of affection. He goes on to suggest that such rituals assist each of us to anticipate our own death more confidently in the knowledge that our dying will be recognised in a similar way. The rituals of mourning feature changes in the appearance of mourners, in terms of wearing appropriate colours, such as black, or items not usually worn, such as hats or armbands. There may be conventions concerning behaviour, such as standing as the cortege passes or driving slowly behind it. The funeral and the wake provide an opportunity for a more social form of support. The duration and expression of mourning may be culturally specified.

Bereavement

For all of us the term 'bereavement' carries a powerful connotation of death, as Osterweis *et al.* emphasise when they define bereavement as 'the fact of loss through death'. Although we must accept this definition, we should bear in mind the other meanings which do not necessarily involve death; perhaps the emphasis in this definition should be on '*the fact of loss*' rather than death.

The other meanings of bereavement become apparent through the etymological evidence. The active verb 'to bereave' means 'to steal anything of value' (Chambers, 1981). From this is derived the well-known and widely-used adjective 'bereft', which is the passive form of the verb and clearly indicates the feelings of the bereaved person following various forms of loss which may be more or less tangible. Both forms are related to the verb 'to reave' (as in the 'border rievers' who were robbers on the English/Scottish border) meaning 'to plunder or rob', again, words which are highly appropriate to describe the feelings of a person who has been bereaved.

Loss

Loss is a term which is widely-used for a number of reasons. The first is that it indicates the 'innocence' or non-contributory involvement of the bereaved person; they have been passive in the event and are suffering through no fault of their own and are deserving of our care and support. The word 'loss' may become particularly helpful in the later stages of grieving when the bereaved person is feeling guilty about any action or inaction on their part which they feel may have contributed to this event.

'Loss' is also a useful word because it is non-specific and may be used in a wide range of situations when grieving is the appropriate response.

This word does not necessarily indicate that a death has occurred, but may suggest that the relationship with a person or an object has been altered in some other way or it may even be appropriate when some part of the body has been removed. I consider some of these other forms of loss later.

On the other hand, it has been suggested that the term 'loss' may be less than helpful because of the connotations which it carries. These may be carried over from its use in other situations when it implies carelessness or irresponsibility in not taking care of one's property and permitting it to 'go missing'. This may be seen to imply that the person who is bereaved is at fault or is to be blamed in another way.

Understanding meanings

The possibility of this adverse interpretation of 'loss' is one example which shows the importance of the words which we may use unthinkingly and which may give rise to hurt in sensitive situations. 'Loss' is an example which clearly demonstrates the need to be thoughtful in our contacts, particularly with those who are bereaved.

There are other, perhaps more hurtful, words which those who are bereaved may encounter in their contacts with midwives and others. As with so many occupational groups, those who work in maternity care have developed their own jargon which serves, among other purposes, to facilitate quick, effective communication among people working under pressure. Unfortunately this jargon may be unthinkingly used in other, non-interprofessional contacts; in these situations their jargon meanings may be less than clear to the lay person, the patient or the parents. Even more seriously, the jargon may carry completely different and possibly negative meanings to the non-professional.

A very appropriate example in this context is the word 'abortion', which carries to lay people the implication of interference ending the pregnancy; to midwives and others this term is value-free in that it means simply that the pregnancy may be ending, for an unspecified reason, before the baby is viable. It is encouraging to observe that more sensitive words such as 'miscarriage' are now used more frequently in this context, although even this term is not devoid of negative connotations (Connolly, 1989a).

Although it is not necessarily hurtful, I avoid the word 'fetus' in this book. This is in recognition of the mother's perception of her developing baby, which by eight to twelve weeks has become to her a real person (Lumley, 1979). The use of words such as fetus are not helpful to communication and may be counterproductive in caring situations.

I use the word 'understanding' to indicate awareness of the issues relating to the experience of bereavement. Thus, it is being used in general terms to reflect our knowledge of this area. Although it may be well-meant, it may not be helpful to say to a person who has been bereaved 'I understand how you are feeling'. This statement, although intended to reassure and comfort, serves to diminish the essentially personal nature of grief. My own experience of a well-intentioned colleague saying this to me when my father died is still disquieting. My recollection of her assumption of similarity between her father's death and that of my father always brings back my feeling of difficulty in communicating with my father and my inability to help him to cope with the last of a long series of difficult experiences.

Meaning and caring

When considering the most appropriate way to describe the feelings and experience of the mother whose baby has died or has been lost in some other way, we should contemplate the words which we use to describe this mother. Long gone are the days when we described mothers in terms of 'the forceps in bed 4' or 'the caesarean in room 12', because these terms reduced the mother to little more than her bed or room number and carried no recognition of the *person* occupying that space.

That she *is* a mother is not in doubt and much of our care revolves around helping her, despite having no baby with her, to realise this. Is it appropriate to refer to this woman as 'a grieving mother'? This term is widely and sympathetically used, but we need to question the effect it has on our perception of her. It, perhaps correctly, focuses our attention on what we consider to be the feature of her care which is most deserving of our attention. Unfortunately, though, it ignores the fact that she is a complete person with, simultaneously, a wide range of other feelings and needs.

As Gohlish (1985) showed, the mother has the difficulties and discomforts which many new mothers encounter, such as relationship adjustments, a sore perineum, afterpains or painful breasts, as well as the more difficult task of coping with her loss. It is essential for us to regard this mother as a complete person who has been bereaved and who needs care which takes many forms, and not only help her with her grieving, crucial though that help may be. In advocating the holistic care of this mother, I accept that we are all too often accused of ignoring the emotional and spiritual aspects of care. On this occasion, however, I find that I am reversing the usual plea and recommend that the physical and practical aspects of this mother's care are given their due attention.

Healthy grieving

In the context of dying and death the concept of a 'good death' is becoming recognised (Kalish, 1985). The value of this concept is not easy to assess because it is widely criticised on the grounds that it merely protects the user from the painful reality of loss by distancing or by intellectualising what is an essentially emotional experience. Despite this criticism, I suggest that the early stages of healthy grieving may be facilitated by appropriate care.

Grieving has been shown to involve the development of the emotional state from the initial numbing impact of learning of the loss through to the point where memories may be recalled with equanimity. The role of the midwife is to help the mother to begin this process of adjusting to the situation in which she finds herself. While accepting that bereavement cannot be regarded as anything other than painful, the midwife is in a position to enable the mother to create memories which she will be able to recall with some degree of satisfaction, in the sense of being able to bring to mind events around the birth and conclude 'Yes, we did that right' or 'I'm glad we were able to do that for my baby' or 'I can look back now and know I was happy with most of the care I received' (Gayton, 1991).

In her care the midwife is able to establish the foundations of healthy grieving, which will end, in due course, with the resolution of the mother's grief and the associated personal growth. The mother will eventually come to realise that her loss has a less negative side. Additionally, as Parkes (1972) observed, 'The experience of grieving can strengthen and bring maturity to those who have been protected from misfortune'.

Grief work

Current thinking about grieving began with the work of Lindemann (1944) in the USA. This unprecedented study followed a tragic fire in the Cocoanut Grove night club and Clark (1991) maintains that it was Lindemann who first introduced the term 'grief work', to indicate that grieving is not static, but an active process in which the ability of the person to complete their task is a major factor affecting the duration of their grief.

Stages of grieving

The model of grieving described by Kubler-Ross (1970) introduced *stages* of grieving, based on her work with people facing death. These well-known and generally-accepted stages feature:

(1) denial or isolation
(2) confusion or anger
(3) bargaining

(4) depression

(5) acceptance.

The concept of stages is valuable in that it emphasises the dynamic nature of grieving and the active role of the bereaved person.

Kubler-Ross built on the work of Lindemann by describing the process in more easily-manageable sections. A serious disadvantage is that this descriptive concept may become prescriptive if a 'professional' considers that grieving 'ought' to progress in a certain sequence. This may give rise to unnecessary and counter-productive anxiety. Such a prescriptive approach also has the potential for limiting individual expression. Wisely, few who have studied and written about grieving have specified the duration of normal grief.

A general pattern

What may be called a 'general pattern' of grieving is common to the various models described in the literature. Each researcher or author, though, emphasises different aspects, depending on the sample of people on whom they focused (the bereaved or the dying) and the intended audience (producing a more or less complex model). We need to approach the concept of a 'general pattern' with caution. It is not possible to assume that those involved in the research studies from which this pattern is drawn were representative of all grieving people or that the findings are invariably generalised.

The immediate reaction

The immediate reaction comprises a temporary defence mechanism consisting essentially of delaying tactics which serve to insulate the bereaved person from the unacceptable reality (Engel, 1961). This gives them time to rally their emotional resources in preparation for their ultimate realisation. Their delaying tactics eventually end and the bereaved person begins to accept the reality of their loss. Bodily symptoms such as sighing respirations may be evident.

This first stage has been described in various ways. Jones (1989) explains it in terms of shock, suggesting a physiological response with or without psychological connotations and the possibility of pathological developments. Kubler-Ross assumed a more purely psychological approach when she described this first stage as denial. In his account of searching for the one who is lost, Parkes emphasises the need of the bereaved person to protect themselves from the awful reality and implies the tentative movement towards the acceptance of that reality.

Developing awareness

Gradually developing awareness (Engel, 1961) manifests itself and with the dawning realisation of the loss come the initial, powerful emotional responses. Guilt, associated with dissatisfaction with unfinished business, may be a major feature. Anger directed at a wide range of probably innocent people demonstrates a partial awareness of the reality of the loss. The need to search for the one who is lost reflects the preoccupation with the *physical* absence of the lost person (Stroebe & Stroebe, 1987). This search may be aggravated by perceptions involving various senses, which may be known as hallucinations, indicating the presence of the person who is lost. Examples would include the mother feeling her baby moving within her or her baby crying. Bargaining permits a gradual, controlled realisation combined with excuse-making in an attempt to rationalise the loss.

As each of these emotional responses is found to be a less than adequate solution it gives way to aimlessness, despondency and apathy which has been termed 'disorganisation' (Bowlby, 1961) and which heralds the onset of the ultimate despair associated with complete recognition of the loss.

Full realisation

Full realisation is demonstrated by the profound depression mentioned by Jones, Kubler-Ross and Parkes. Feelings of loss may be transferred onto the body of the bereaved person in the form of feelings of incompleteness or bodily mutilation, such as the 'great emptiness' mentioned by a widow (Parkes, 1976). This depression brings with it psychological changes, such as poor concentration and difficulty in sleeping, as well as bodily problems such as those affecting the gastro-intestinal tract.

Resolution

The final stage of grieving is resolution, which is said to have been achieved when the bereaved person is able to remember comfortably, realistically and with equanimity the pleasures and disappointments of their lost relationship (Chaney, 1981). Kubler-Ross describes this stage in relatively passive terms as acceptance, whereas Parkes describes the more active processes of recovery, reorganisation and reintegration.

The potential for long-term personal benefit associated with bereavement is suggested in the account of the resolution stage given by Jones. He looks forward to the new identity assumed by the bereaved person, incorporating all that has been learned from the experience of bereavement, including the inevitable personal growth and development as well as the valuing of others' support, both of which permit an increased ability to cope with other, unknown crises yet to be faced.

Variations between individuals

As people oscillate and hesitate between stages (Stroebe & Stroebe,

1987), variations between individuals in the duration and progress of grieving may be recognised. Parkes summarises the tendency towards sequential recovery through the emergence of succeeding stages: 'Grief is not a set of symptoms which start after a loss and then gradually fade away. It involves a succession of clinical pictures which blend into and replace one another.'

Pathological forms of grief

In the same way as accounts of the stages of grieving vary, so do descriptions of the complicated or otherwise pathological forms of grief. The pathological forms of grief are usually described as involving deviations in the severity of grieving and/or its duration. This observation applies to the account by Parkes which focused on the time-related aspects. On this occasion he described prolonged grieving which may occur separately from or in conjunction with delayed grieving. Lindemann provided a valuable account of what he identified as 'morbid grief reactions'. He first described temporal deviations in terms of delay in beginning grieving. He then went on to detail the 'distorted' reactions including:

(1) overactivity without sense of loss
(2) hypochondriasis, involving developing the symptoms of the person who is lost
(3) genuine psychosomatic disorders
(4) changed relationships
(5) furious hostility
(6) schizophrenic picture
(7) withdrawal from the community and loss of social interaction
(8) behaviour detrimental to the person's own social and economic existence
(9) agitated depression.

Parkes mentions what appears to be a voluntary or deliberate deviation from the usual pattern when he details 'excessive avoidance of grieving'. This is clearly a form of delayed grieving, but it is a form in which the bereaved person assumes control over the timing of their grief. Parkes goes on to describe chronic grieving and also the condition termed 'hypochondriasis' by Lindemann.

Rynearson (1987) criticises the 'oversimplistic' view of pathological grief assumed by Lindemann and others who followed in his footsteps. Rynearson suggests that carers should focus on not just the person's current grieving, but also the events which preceded the grief and even the loss. That is, it may be necessary to take account of the relationship between the bereaved person and the one for whom they are grieving.

Rynearson suggests three categories of dysfunctional grief response:

- **Dependent grief syndrome** involves an imbalanced relationship in which the bereaved person has been and continues to be clinging and over-reliant on the person who is lost.
- **Unexpected loss syndrome** follows a sudden loss and perpetuates the initial shock and denial in a long-term withdrawn anxiety state.
- **Conflicted grief syndrome** is associated with an insecure or ambivalent relationship, the uncertainty of which may delay the onset of grieving.

Rynearson explains how this approach to pathological forms of grief may be utilised in the care of people with dysfunctional grieving. This approach serves to emphasise, in this context, that the midwife and other carers should avoid making assumptions about the relationship of the mother and baby and that grieving will follow a prescribed pattern. Such assumptions may not, according to Rynearson, facilitate grieving.

Unique features of perinatal loss

As briefly mentioned already, any form of loss presents difficulties in adjustment, but loss around the time of birth carries with it certain problems which may serve to confound the progress of healthy grieving. As midwives we must be especially aware of the possibility of these problems and intervene appropriately to prevent their occurrence and facilitate grieving.

The horror, which death and loss inevitably carry with them, may be particularly difficult for the new mother. Being young, her experience of previous loss, if any, is limited. For some mothers, their adolescent adjustments are barely completed; even less have they acquired the maturity needed to come to terms with loss and death (Bourne, 1979). This sense of horror is aggravated by the largely appropriate emphasis our society places on the healthiness or normality of childbirth. While generally focusing on the physiological nature of childbearing, little attention is given to the possibility of what may be known as reproductive failure. This serves to increase the mother's difficulty in accepting the situation when it arises.

In spite of the prevalent perception of the normality of childbearing, it remains imbued with some magical, almost mystical qualities. This awe is often impressed on me by mothers admiring their newborn babies who ask 'Did she really come out of me?' It may be that the removal of childbirth from the domestic setting to the hospital has served to increase this sense of wonder and to hinder the acceptance of any deviation in this process.

The bewilderment that follows the simultaneous occurrence of new life and death relates to the general assumption that there will be a life-span, traditionally three score years and ten, separating the two events. When new life and death appear to become fused together, our entire perception of the world may be called into question. As Bourne (1979) states 'the experience becomes one that stands reality on its head'.

If the baby has some unexpected kind of malformation, the mother may encounter even greater difficulty in recognising the baby to whom she has given birth as the one she had been expecting. This may cause particular problems if the mother had assumed that the battery of prenatal tests had given her baby a 'clean bill of health'.

The difficulties experienced by those caring for the mother may aggravate her difficulty in coming to terms with her loss. Those who come into midwifery assuming it to be a happy area of care, become profoundly shocked when they realise that this is not invariably so. Their sense of having failed the mother may impede their ability to share or at least listen to her expression of her feelings of loss. The response of the staff to perinatal loss is implicit in the care of this mother and may be manifested in apparently well-meaning help, such as single accommodation in the maternity unit and early transfer home (Hughes, 1987). The extent to which the emotional responses of staff affect their ability to provide appropriate care is discussed in Chapter 9.

The social support, shown by Clark to be essential to healthy grieving, may be less easily available to the mother who miscarries or gives birth to a stillborn baby, because her baby was not known to others near her. Grandparents' expectations of their grandchild, for example, may help them to offer some sympathy, but not the depth of feeling shared over the loss of a known and loved person. This problem applies to a lesser extent to the partner of the mother who is bereaved and to a greater extent if the loss occurs earlier in pregnancy (Raphael, 1984a).

The development of the relationship

Certain processes which happen near the time of the birth mould the mother's relationship with her baby and, therefore, their significance to loss and grief cannot be overstated. These processes and the loving relationship which ensues are fundamental to our understanding of loss, and grief is the price which we all must pay for our experience of loving.

Attachment

Developmentally the human being is so immature at birth that the baby depends on care by others for survival. How this care and, hence, the survival of humanity is ensured has long been a topic for speculation. Our thinking has moved on since Freud's psychoanalytical ideas and his assumption that human babies have innate biological drives, such as hunger, which demand gratification. The behaviourists' ideas followed, but they focused on attachment developing through reinforcement of learning. In the 1960s their biological explanations were modified when external factors, such as touch, were found to affect the mother–child relationship (Harlow & Harlow, 1966).

Simultaneously, ethology (the study of animals in their natural habitat) added imprinting to our understanding of the mother–child relationship. This is the process by which, typically, a newly-hatched duck assumes the first moving object it sees to be its source of comfort and security; this object would ordinarily be its mother or 'primary caregiver'. The limited time-span for imprinting gives us the 'critical' or 'sensitive period' (Mussen *et al.*, 1990).

Bowlby (1958) integrated ethology with psychoanalytical principles to support his thesis that attachment derives from neither drive-reduction nor prior learning. He argued that a human newborn is programmed to emit signals or behaviours which will keep caregivers near enough to meet the newborn's needs and ensure survival.

Attachment according to Bretherton (1987) is 'A regulatory system hypothesised to exist within a person ... to regulate behaviors that maintain proximity to and contact with a discriminated protective person, referred to as the attachment figure. From the psychological vantage point of the attached person, however, the system's set goal is felt security'. Newborn behaviours initiate and maintain secure attachment to the caregiver (Brazelton, 1973). Bowlby's thesis (1977) is that attachment derives from the need for security and safety and that the young form enduring attachments with a limited number of individuals.

The role of attachment in healthy development lies in its provision of a secure base from which a child is able to explore the physical and psychological surroundings, and to which the child may retreat if threats become overwhelming (Bowlby, 1979:137).

Attachment and loss

Attachment is significant in relation to perinatal loss because grieving is the inevitable eventual corollary of any warm, loving relationship. These two contrasting aspects of attachment became apparent in Bowlby's research with toddlers separated from their mothers by the unusual situation of being admitted to residential care. His research identified a characteristic biphasic response involving protest, despair, unresponsiveness and tantrums. It became apparent that the absence of the attachment object meant that the secure base no longer existed, engendering terror of the unknown. Bowlby (1979) equates adult grief with separation anxiety, when the security of a loved person and relationship is lost, leaving a frighteningly incomprehensible void.

Bonding

Bonding as a topic generates more heat than light. It is the first preliminary stage in the events which lead to attachment (Mussen *et al.*, 1990). The plethora of research in this area has been associated with many changes in our care of the new mother and baby. Whether these changes are necessarily for the benefit of the mother–infant dyad is questionable (Herbert & Sluckin, 1985:123). Considerable attention has been given to early postnatal bonding because it equates with the 'love at first sight' which has commonly been assumed to be fundamental to mother-love, but events during pregnancy may be more significant in the context of perinatal loss.

Changes in pregnancy

Traditionally we have assumed that the mother did not begin to experience maternal love until she laid eyes on her baby (Morrin, 1983). Hence, only recently has there been research into how the mother comes to relate to her baby prenatally.

On the basis of interviews with 20 mothers whose newborn babies had died, Kennell *et al.* (1970) were able to conclude that an affectionate mother–child relationship was present by the time the baby was due to be born. As many of the mothers had had no visual or tactile contact with their babies, any postnatal stimuli to affection were excluded.

Grace (1989) measured the way in which the mother's affection for her child develops, showing the mother's increasingly positive feelings as pregnancy progresses. Similar instruments were used to study the effects of maternal age, the experience of quickening and the physical symptoms of pregnancy on the developing relationship in 80 pregnant mothers (Lerum & Lobiondo-Wood, 1989). These researchers found that only quickening has any effect on the relationship, and that is positive. The effects of ultrasound scans, which have been said to enhance the relationship, were unclear, but those mothers who were well-supported showed a high level of attachment.

Unlike the two previous studies, Zeanah *et al.* (1990) based their study of the prenatal mother–baby relationship on the mother's interpretation of fetal movements. Mothers were shown to have sufficiently clear ideas about their baby's temperament during pregnancy to complete a questionnaire anticipating how the baby would react in given circumstances. It is impossible to judge whether the mother's interpretations of fetal behaviour derive from her own fantasies or from the actual movements, but the researchers correctly relate her interpretation to the developing relationship.

In her qualitative study, Stainton (1990) sought 26 couples' impressions of their unborn babies in the third trimester. She identified four different levels of awareness, coexisting simultaneously. In ascending order, these are as follows:

- idea of the baby
- awareness of the baby's presence
- awareness of the baby's specific behaviours
- awareness of the baby's interactive ability.

These interpretations of fetal behaviour suggest that knowledge of the psychosocial interaction with the unborn baby may have implications for our care of childbearing women in the same way as the more widely-used objective assessments because, Stainton reminds us, a stronger mother–baby relationship during pregnancy facilitates postnatal mothering.

The limited benefits of ultrasound scans on the developing relationship in comparison with quickening are shown by Reading (1989). Lumley (1990) endorses these points and raises other disconcerting questions about routine investigations.

As our knowledge of the mother–baby relationship during pregnancy is still so limited, attempts to influence its development are inappropriate. There is little doubt, though, that the strength of the mother's relationship with her unborn baby results in her need to grieve if the baby is lost.

Postnatal bonding

The research project which is best-known and has probably had the greatest influence on our care of the newborn and her mother is the work by Klaus *et al.* (1972). Their experimental study was undertaken against a background of restricted mother–baby contact in USA maternity units. The control group of 14 mothers was permitted the usual contact with their babies, that is, 30 minutes at feeding five times daily. The experiment or extended contact group of 14 mothers cuddled their naked babies in bed with them for an extra five hours on each of their three days in hospital. Observations and interviews were made at one month and one year.

Findings of differences between the two groups were emphasised, although there were many similarities. During a paediatric examination, the extended contact group showed greater reluctance to leave their babies and extended contact mothers responded more to their babies' crying and maintained greater eye-to-eye contact during feeds. These researchers concluded that extended contact was necessary for bonding; others went as far as to suggest that without this contact adverse outcomes, such as child abuse, were more likely. Thus, bonding theory evolved into dogma or 'bonding doctrine' (Herbert & Sluckin, 1985; Sluckin *et al.*, 1983).

This study has influenced our care for the better; the requirement for the baby to be in the postnatal ward within ten minutes of birth disappeared. In another unit midwives were, briefly, required to record whether a mother had 'bonded' with her baby in the birthing room. Negative observations brought social work intervention.

Whether the changes in our practice are justified by the results of the Klaus *et al.* study continues to be questioned on methodological grounds. Observer bias was a problem. But it is hard to envisage how a 'blind' study of attachment could be designed; as mothers and carers *must* know which group a mother is in and be influenced in their behaviour and observations respectively (Schaffer, 1977). The sample comprised disadvantaged mothers in whom any intervention might have improved the outcome.

These researchers' use of biological terms to explain their conclusions, such as the 'sensitive period', ignored current knowledge of the complexity of mother–child interactions and the uniquely human social organisation. The sensitive period is implausible in humans, due to maternal mortality and morbidity requiring 'adoption' by other carers in the former and longer and more variable attachment periods in the latter (Richards, 1983).

In demolishing the bonding doctrine, Sluckin *et al.* (1983) state that bonding publicity may engender excessively high expectations in the mother. Failure to achieve any part of the doctrine leaves her disappointed with her experience and, more important, anxious about her ability to relate to her new baby. Unrealistic expectations may be prevented by informing mothers of recent research evidence which questions the instantaneous all-or-nothing phenomenon (Dunn, 1975; de Chateau, 1980; Leifer *et al.*, 1972; Grossman *et al.*, 1981).

The perfect baby

The baby on which the mother focuses her fantasies during pregnancy is the baby she comes to love at that time and who she may eventually need to grieve. This baby's image is a composite of those she loves and admires, including herself, partner, parents and other children. If she has no children already, she will base her fantasies on what she learns from other parents and from the media. As well as helping her to form a relationship with her baby, this process enables her to work through old conflicts, especially any concerning her relationship with her own mother (Solnit & Stark, 1961). Inevitably the mother's fantasies involve wishing for and dreaming of a perfect baby, but lurking in the background is the fear of a baby being born with a disability.

Solnit and Stark state that there is usually some discrepancy between the mother's fantasies and her actual baby; she may have expected her baby to have more hair, or be surprised at how long her baby spends awake, or perhaps she had not expected to use quite so many nappies. The mother's narcissistic investment in her fantasy baby (see Chapter 3) may aggravate the discrepancy between the two babies. Disentangling this discrepancy and accepting the real baby is one of the developmental tasks involved in becoming a mother.

The fantasy baby is explained by Lewis (1976 & 1979a) as her 'inside baby' in contrast to her 'outside baby' for whom she must care. Lewis describes the perplexing sense of loss which a mother ordinarily experiences at losing her inside baby, but she is consoled by the presence of her outside baby. The effort required of the mother to match up her fantasy baby to her real baby is neither easy nor spontaneous (Raphael-Leff, 1991:310) and may account for some mothers' overwhelming indifference on first seeing the baby.

The mother's expectations of both her baby and her experience of birth may give her at least momentary cause for regret. Dissatisfaction may relate to internal factors or to those outwith her control. She may similarly regret that the baby is the wrong sex (Kowalski, 1987).

Thus, even in normal childbearing there exists an element of regret. The mother may feel the loss of the fantasy baby to whom she did not give birth, for the baby of the 'right' gender who was not born or for the hoped-for birth experience which did not happen. These losses require the mother to grieve and may assume the proportions of a bereavement (Parrish, 1980). It may be difficult for others to understand why a mother with an apparently ideal outcome has moments of sorrow. She may find it hard to acknowledge, even to herself. The mother needs our help to articulate and come to terms with her loss in the same way as any loss is eventually resolved.

Summary

The need of the grieving mother for expert help and support in emotional, psychological and physical terms may be illustrated by an analogy first used by Engel (1961). He compared the psychological trauma involved in grief with the physical trauma of a cut to the skin. He explained how healing is necessary for both forms of trauma to enable the body and mind to regain their usual balance or homeostasis. The degree of help needed to achieve healing varies, depending on a number of factors. Minor abrasions will normally heal spontaneously, without any outside intervention, but major wounds require extra assistance. The major psychological trauma of grief following perinatal loss may also require assistance.

Even in the experiences of childbearing which we regard as ideal, when a satisfied mother produces a healthy baby, there may be an element of regret, giving rise to the need to grieve. Grief is 'the other side of the coin' of the loving relationship which develops during pregnancy. Because the mother's relationship is with an idealised fantasy baby, postnatally she may need to grieve for not having fulfilled her fantasies and achieved her expectations.

The midwife has the earliest opportunity to provide assistance for the mother who is grieving either a baby lost through death or a baby whose image needs readjusting. It is to be hoped that the midwife also has the knowledge and skill to care for both of these mothers.

Chapter 2
Researching Perinatal Loss: Problems, Dangers and Opportunities

To begin this chapter I look at the need for research and the use we make of research-based knowledge. The inherent problems of researching perinatal grief are discussed next. Then, having already considered our use of research, I look at its misuse; to do this I focus on examples of research becoming dogma, which we find in areas relating to grief and which raise fundamental issues. Finally, I look at how to avoid such rigidity by focusing on my recent study (Mander, 1992d), identifying a relevant research framework and highlighting outstanding research needs.

Do we need research?

As with any research problem, I begin with a question. Here, as I asked the midwives in my recent study (see below), I ask: 'How do we know how to care for the grieving mother?' The answers emphasised experience; many informants cited examples of their own childbearing and their occupational experience (Mander, 1992b). These midwives also recounted the limited contribution of formal methods of learning, such as lectures, refresher courses and reading journals. While recognising the importance of experience, including continuing education, to knowledgeable effective care, a questioning attitude to proposed and existing practices is a crucial precursor (Chalmers, 1993). It may even be our *duty* to question established practice (Davis, 1983). The responses to my enquiry (above) indicate the preparedness of midwives to question their practice:

Izzy I always do my utmost to care as best I can. Care is really quite well done. I have never had any negative feedback. Really, I've not had very much contact afterwards at all.

Gay I haven't had any training at all to help me to look after these mothers. . . . I think that the care that we give is quite reasonable. We give the mothers support and help and advice.

Annie My ideas are my ideas, I don't know whether they are necessarily correct.

Ginnie I often feel frustrated that I don't know what more I can do for them.
Nellie We try our best to give them as much time to talk to us as possible. But I
feel that really that isn't as good as we should be doing.

As the comments by Ginnie and Nellie show, a questioning attitude may manifest itself when contemplating day-to-day practice. This may be supported by critical reading, the appropriate use of research and, possibly, doing research. The reality of research utilisation was noted by the Health Committee who observed maternity care's limited research base (House of Commons, 1992):

> 'Too many fashionable interventions . . . have been introduced without evaluation either of cost–benefit ratios or the reactions of women who undergo them.'

Is midwives' care of the grieving mother founded on 'fashionable interventions'? Does our care constitute an unplanned, uncontrolled and unrecognised experiment? We should closely examine our care of the grieving mother and the knowledge on which it is founded.

The development of research into perinatal grief

The knowledge-base which we use to care for the grieving mother originated with Freud (1917/59), who likened grief to a 'painful wound'. This dispensed with the Judaeo–Christian view of grief, which regarded it as an unnecessary and unhelpful luxury; mourners were urged to avoid 'fruitless and unavailing grief' (Pine & Brauer, 1986). Freud, whose ideas were clinically-derived, moved us closer to therapeutic support of the bereaved.

Lindemann was the first to systematically observe grief (Prior, 1993; Lindemann, 1944). His, admittedly opportunistic, study sampled 101 people affected by the disastrous Cocoanut Grove night club fire. Lindemann's conclusions relating to the nature of grief failed to make allowance for the complex relationships between the bereaved and the deceased (Rynearson, 1987). His tunnel vision reminds us to avoid assumptions about others' grief based on personal value systems.

Despite being founded on the unusual sample of children facing separation by institutionalisation, Bowlby's ideas (1979) moved grieving theory forward, by demonstrating fundamental links between attachment and grief. He hypothesised that without loving attachment, there can be no loss. Thus, grief is the price that human beings pay for the joy of loving; often known as 'the cost of commitment'.

Bowlby's ideas are closely and powerfully linked with those of Parkes (1976), though their research populations were at opposite extremes of the age range. Parkes, as have others (Stroebe & Stroebe, 1987), researched the grief of widows; but unlike previous researchers, Parkes was able to demonstrate the contribution of the wider social community by showing us the value of relatively 'low-tech' interventions, such as bereavement counselling. The significance of counselling is reinforced by his observation of the widespread and harmful effects of the stigma of loss, which may result in social isolation of the bereaved.

Parkes' ideas were utilised by Forrest *et al.* (1982) when they researched support and counselling after perinatal bereavement. They, like Parkes, emphasise the long-term counselling of the family, compared with the supportive midwifery interventions at the birth and death. In an experimental design involving 50 mothers of babies who had died perinatally, half of the mothers received 'ideal' supported care, while the 'contrast' group received care of the usual variable standard.

The supported group were encouraged to see, hold and name their dead baby. The baby was photographed. The mother chose, whenever possible, where she was cared for and her transfer home was unhurried. Bereavement counselling was offered to both parents within two days of the loss. While the counselled mothers recovered from their grief more quickly than the contrast group, by the 14-month assessment there was no significant difference between the two groups.

These findings are largely reassuring, though it may be that the intervention served only to speed the grief of the supported group. It is necessary to wonder, apart from the pain enduring, whether marginally longer grief automatically reflects less effective grief. The significance of the high drop-out rate from the supported group is another cause for concern (see Chapter 5).

Issues arising out of previous research

The gestation or age at which the baby is lost has received much research attention (Pine & Brauer, 1986). This relates to either the assumption of the unseen being ungrieved or to our increasing understanding of how the emotional relationship develops during pregnancy (see Chapter 1).

Contrary to traditional assumptions, parents of newborns who die have been found to grieve more successfully than bereaved parents of older children (Murray & Callan, 1988). On the other hand, an authoritative study showed that there are no significant differences between the grief of women losing their babies through miscarriage, stillbirth or neonatal death (Peppers & Knapp, 1980). Despite such research, the grief of the mother who miscarries is still denigrated. An example is the diktat by Bourne and Lewis (1991) that 'people should not be pushed into magnifying miscarriage'. Rather than magnifying or denigrating any mother's grief, we should accept the loss for what it means to her.

The effects on family relationships have attracted research attention, focusing mainly on differences in grieving between mother and father and any ensuing disharmony (Klass, 1986). I consider the implications for fathers and couples in Chapter 6. The serious deficit in research-based knowledge into the effects of perinatal loss on siblings is well-recognised (Leon, 1990:193; Borg & Lasker, 1982). The research by Dyregrov (1988, 1991) illuminates sibling reactions to perinatal loss (Chapter 6). This has helped to fill the void, although a retrospective view, uncertainty about the therapy/research orientation and reliance on mothers' accounts of the sibling's loss limit its value.

By predicting and measuring grief, attempts have been made to identify those most at risk of disordered grieving and to evaluate helpful interventions. Predictors were sought among 130 parents who had experienced perinatal loss by using a self-administered questionnaire (Murray & Callan, 1988). This obtained, as well as demographic data, features of the loss, levels of professional support and psychological well-being.

Like Benfield *et al.* (1978) and Peppers and Knapp (1980), these researchers found that better supported parents grieved more healthily, lending weight to the usual assumption that those who are less supported face worse outcomes. Like others, however, these researchers also made the mistake of focusing on professional interventions and ignoring the grieving parents' social support system. It may be that the holistic view ordinarily adopted by midwives makes us ideally suited to research the social effects. The development of a grief scoring system has been shown to be useful (Benfield *et al.*, 1978; Kennell *et al.*, 1970), although its clinical uses are less clear.

Criticisms of care inevitably arise when bereaved mothers are asked to recount their experiences. For all mothers we must take these criticisms seriously; although we may wonder, for those interviewed while actively grieving, whether they are still deciding who to blame.

In her retrospective study of 15 mothers who had experienced perinatal loss, Hermione Lovell *et al.* (1986) found that mothers sensed the limited time staff were able or willing to spend with them. She also found that the community midwives' visits were variably appreciated. The medical checks six weeks postnatally were well-attended but under-utilised, being of a merely physical orientation. This observation may be related to a phenomenon identified in a study of 22 mothers who had experienced perinatal loss (Alice Lovell, 1983); the difficulty staff feel in coping with death may prevent them from supporting the mother. This researcher also emphasises the limited social support offered to the grieving mother by the so-called community.

In my study (Mander, 1992d) many of the relinquishing mothers were critical of certain aspects of their care; I have termed these experiences 'cockups'. Like other mothers, Jessica had been told not to have any

contact with her baby; unfortunately this message was not commu-
nicated to all the staff caring for her:

Jessica   Just after the baby was born I was in a room with all the other mothers.
He was in my arms for about an hour. There was some kind of mix up,
because when my parents came in at night he had been brought out to me
again. By that time I had been put in a side room by myself. I had him that
night and I was quite happy with myself. The next day the nurses said that
was it! I couldn't have any more contact! Then one of the midwives said to
me 'That bond hasn't got to be there. You can't bond. You can't see him
any more'.

As well as raising bonding issues which I explore later, this example
shows that faulty communication between staff leaves the mother
feeling uncertain.

Midwifery research has been shown to be undervalued by midwives
themselves (Hicks, 1992). In a small and questionably ethical study,
Hicks shows that midwives rate a research report significantly higher if
they believe it is written by a medical practitioner rather than a midwife.
Hicks concludes that research is not perceived as being essential to
midwifery, but she neglects the prevailing value system. The accuracy of
Hicks' observation is endorsed by the reception of two midwifery studies
on perinatal grief. The study by Hughes (1986, 1987), on the location
of the mother's care, has been denigrated (Adams & Prince, 1990) and
ignored. Gohlish's study (1985) on the nursing behaviours helpful to the
bereaved mother has been shown by my own research to be unknown
among midwives.

Methodological issues

There are certain issues which are particularly important in the planning, reading, evaluation and utilisation of research into perinatal loss.

That '*careless research* is as immoral as careless surgery' is argued by
Davis (1983). His example of good research comprising the wise and
correct use of statistics, leads us to suspect that quantitative research is
invariably good. Although terms such as 'bad' research are bandied
about, they may mean little more than 'research methods which I have
not used and don't understand'. Such deprecatory terms may be used by
researchers to describe others' work, when their insecurity with
unknown methods underpins the difficulty. Truly immoral research is
that done at some cost to the respondents and the funding body, but
which is never reported or disseminated to practitioners (Hicks, 1993).

The *design* of many grief research projects is criticised for using a
retrospective approach, inevitably relying on recall. A grief-stricken
memory is likely to distort the data and result in bias. The longitudinal

prospective study is a valuable alternative, which may provide accurate current data, but unfortunately a time lapse may be necessary to allow the bereaved mother to recover from the worst pain of her grief (Leon, 1990:189; Oglethorpe, 1989; Stroebe & Stroebe, 1987).

The *sample* should be selected to minimise risks to subjects, such as causing pain or impairing grieving. As always, the sample size should be the smallest number possible consistent with being suitably representative (Davis, 1983).

The *response rate* indicates the acceptability and importance which the members of the population attach to the research. A low response rate raises questions of whether those who did not respond differ significantly from those who did (Atkinson, 1991). In grief research we expect the response rate to be low compared with other topics (Stroebe & Stroebe, 1987), but my observation is that in most studies the response is nearer to Cooper's (1980) 66% than Benfield's (1978) 27%. Obviously, this reflects only those studies which actually state the response rate; this information is all too often omitted. Leon (1990) reminds us of the risk of 'attenuation' of the sample, as in the study by Forrest *et al.* (1982), which reduces the possibility of statistically significant findings.

The *representativeness* of the sample may be hampered by the nature of the study, as those who agree to be involved may be grieving atypically. Perhaps it is only those whose grief is progressing smoothly who agree to participate, or, alternatively, those needing more help who hope to get it through involvement in research (Stroebe & Stroebe, 1987)?

The *location* of a suitable sample is addressed by Worden (1992), who discusses the diverse social groupings and distances which a researcher may need to cover. The random nature of grief means that the sample must be, like Lindemann's (1944), an opportunistic or convenience sample, reducing the researcher's control over the study. Discussing future research into perinatal loss, Leon (1990) emphasises the problem of finding a suitable sample when so many potentially different forms of loss are included.

Researching grief brings certain unique problems. Particularly likely is the Hawthorne effect, when the person's behaviour changes because of their research involvement (Stroebe & Stroebe, 1987). Such a change clearly invalidates the data. Worden (1992) focuses on problems associated with measuring grief by using health as an indicator, as Winkler and van Keppel (1984) did in their study of relinquishing mothers. Proxy measures may be used, as these may be more accessible than health data; examples include medication, general practitioner (GP) contacts or hospital admission. Symptoms are, thus, inappropriately regarded as manifestations of grief, whereas these 'health behaviours' are even more culture-bound and socially-determined than grief itself. Leon (1990) observes that treatment may be more closely related to help-seeking variables than to the person's degree of disturbance. It may be that medication is the least reliable proxy for grief, as the values of the prescriber also contribute.

The danger of dogma

I have considered already the reasons why research-based knowledge is crucial to improve our care of the grieving mother and the benefits which accrue. Because examples of less beneficial effects of research arise in our care, it is necessary to look at the potential for harm. By this I mean research findings having been elevated to the level of strict dogma which, by definition, one questions at one's peril.

The first example of research being used to justify dogma is found in what Herbert and Sluckin (1985) call the 'bonding doctrine', resulting in mothers being harassed when they are least able to question their care. History demonstrates the plethora of child-care gurus, such as Truby-King, whose ideas have initially required adherence, have subsequently been challenged and eventually rejected. Unlike the instantaneous, cataclysmic, all-or-nothing 'gluing', as it is all too often presented, the mother–baby relationship grows gradually, through learning to know and coming to understand each other. There are clearly certain factors which hinder this relationship from developing, as there are others which facilitate it.

Another example of research being elevated to dogma is even more closely related to our present topic (Lewis & Bourne, 1989). The danger is that certain forms of care may be applied universally as a panacea to 'solve' the mother's grief (Bourne & Lewis, 1991); examples include the formerly widespread recommendation of 'have another' (see Chapter 12) and the current vogue for visual and tactile maternal–child contact. These authors suggest that many interventions may be effective only in the short-term. Their disregard for recommendations for caring for the mother who miscarries (SANDS, 1991) ignores research emphasising the grief of miscarriage (Peppers & Knapp, 1980) and questioning the value of contact (Cooper, 1980); we are reminded of the shaky foundation on which our current care of the mother experiencing perinatal loss is built (Leon, 1990).

A third way in which dogma becomes significant in the context of research into perinatal loss is in the design of the research. Those who are responsible for approving access for research, the 'gatekeepers', encounter difficulty understanding research which incorporates ideas or methods with which they are not acquainted. For this reason they may be wary of approving research proposals which are incongruent with their attitudes to 'patients' or with their hard-edged views of research.

In my study, her limited view of the role of the midwife prevented one social worker from co-operating (Mander, 1992c). Another's conviction that grief was a short-term phenomenon had a similar effect. Limited understanding of grieving also became apparent in correspondence with research ethics committees (RECs). Criticisms of the research method related to the flexible nature of my data collection, being equated with 'sociological-type' and, hence, 'bad' research.

For these reasons, I propose that we, as carers, read research critically, use it questioningly and undertake appropriately-designed studies, rather than be vulnerable to the whims of medical or even psychological fashion.

A recent study

In a recent research project, I examined care in a particularly vulnerable group of grieving mothers. The issues raised by the mothers and by those who care for them assist our understanding of perinatal grief. My research developed from observations of the demise of the 'rugger pass' approach to the care of the bereaved mother, involving the speedy removal of her dead baby. It was necessary to learn whether more enlightened approaches to care are also being offered to the mother relinquishing her baby for adoption. I describe here the design of a study undertaken to investigate this issue; methodological issues relating to dogma in research design become apparent.

The research approach

The lack of previous research on midwives' care of the relinquishing mother and its innately sensitive nature, led me to choose a qualitative research approach with some quantitative elements. Qualitative research seeks to understand the event from the perspective of the person experiencing it – the 'emic' approach (Harris, 1968). A holistic picture emerges, demonstrating the interrelatedness and interdependence of differing facets of the event (Leininger, 1985).

Some argue that this approach is 'soft' and 'unscientific'. This is a strength in the present context, because the qualitative approach is well-suited to describing and, thus, understanding the subjective viewpoint of the mother about her relinquishment (Aamodt, 1982; Parse *et al.*, 1985; Van Maanen, 1982).

The advantages of large-scale studies of the effects of grief may be compared with smaller-scale in-depth research (Stroebe & Stroebe, 1987). The epidemiological data collected in the former serve a different purpose from the 'fine-grained' details on matters such as coping strategies gained in the latter. Thus, I had to choose between statistical significance and in-depth insight; the research questions determined my choice. My choice was modified by including both qualitative and quantitative elements to achieve a broader picture through incorporating different research approaches in the research design (Jick, 1983; Denzin, 1970); this further increased the rigour of the data.

The research questions

On the basis of the literature available and my personal experience, six research questions emerged:

(1) What is the experience of the mother relinquishing her baby?
(2) To what extent is the experience of a relinquishing mother in the UK similar to those of mothers in other countries?
(3) How, in the midwife's view, does the care she gives to a relinquishing mother compare with that provided for another mother without a baby?
(4) How are decisions made regarding the midwife's care of the relinquishing mother?
(5) What knowledge is involved in making these decisions?
(6) How is this knowledge acquired?

The method

I planned the fieldwork in three phases, examining the viewpoints of those involved. These were, first, previous relinquishing mothers (who had relinquished a baby in the past), second, experienced midwives and, third, current relinquishing mothers (planning relinquishment).

Phase 1 – Aimed to assess the relevance of other countries' literature on long-term feelings about relinquishment by interviewing mothers who had previously relinquished a baby.
Phase 2 – Aimed to explore midwifery care, with particular reference to whether the care of a relinquishing mother differs from that provided for another mother without a baby. A sample of experienced midwives would be interviewed.
Phase 3 – Aimed to observe and describe the experience of the relinquishing mother using a prospective, longitudinal technique. Interviews with a small group of mothers would focus on the experience of giving birth while making the decision to relinquish her baby. The extent to which midwifery care had helped her through the experience would be sought. Interviews would be held in the women's homes postnatally and some months later.

Obtaining permission for research access

Gaining access to suitable relinquishing mothers and midwives involved obtaining ethical approval and permission from midwife managers, respectively. Because it had been necessary to recruit previous relinquishing mothers from a wide area, I decided to recruit midwives from a similar area. My approaches elicited enthusiastic, sympathetic and helpful support and the managers gave permission for me to seek the midwives' participation. Midwives were given permission to be interviewed during their on-duty time in health board premises, if they wished.

Access to a suitable sample of relinquishing mothers for Phase 1 was unproblematical after contacting birth parents' groups, whose organisers and members were keen to participate (Mander, 1992c). Ethical approval and access for Phase 3 presented major difficulties. Eventually a case-study approach was utilised for the one mother I was able to recruit (Mander, 1992d).

The instrument and personal implications

I used a semi-structured interview format, allowing the informant to control the topics, although my introduction reiterated my area of interest, which I had explained during the initial contact. My frequently-updated interview schedule comprised a list of questions, in addition to which I encouraged the informant to introduce relevant issues. My questions were based on the literature, my occupational and other experience and, in later interviews, issues raised by earlier informants.

An essential feature of this form of fieldwork is the way in which I, the researcher, present and use my personality during the interview (Lipson, 1989). This applies to such an extent that my personality constitutes part of the research instrument, in contrast with the usual need for the researcher to be a neutral 'non-person' to avoid bias.

The researcher must be conscious of any intuitive or personal reactions to the informant or information gathered (Field & Morse, 1987). Examples include my revulsion when Francesca recounted the activities of her peers in an alien subculture, or sorrow at Quelia's pathetically limited outlook on life, or overwhelming feelings of identification due to a common early post-war working-class background with Barbara and Debra.

In her, not dissimilar, research into single mothers' decision-making, Macintyre (1975) noted the benefits of perceived shared views for recruitment and data collection. Her informants felt more willing to talk to her because they regarded her as young, and would have been less open with an older woman or man. This was linked with an assumption that she would 'know how they felt' without being too involved. As Macintyre observes, however, she does not know whether some mothers may have perceived these attributes as reasons for *not* participating. Clearly, assumptions of empathy on the part of the researcher do not help the research. By being aware of such reactions we are able to take account of them in both the fieldwork and the analysis of the data.

For the researcher, emotional discomfort may follow such personal involvement (Freilich, 1979). One of the RECs questioned how I would cope with the emotional impact of undertaking a study involving such powerful feelings. This may be through a supporting team of researchers who are able to share problems (Lipson, 1989); but for this study this was impossible and I relied on domestic and social support.

The emotional toll which research takes is particularly significant in qualitative studies, where personal involvement with the work, if not the informants, is crucial. This point is rarely raised, as even Lipson's perceptive and sympathetic work mentions only the effects on the study, rather than on the researcher.

Gans (1982), however, does consider the effects of involvement on the researcher; he recommends that the researcher should, early on in the study, take a long hard look at their emotional vulnerability. In order to continue, they need to work out, perhaps with the help of a counsellor, whether their anxieties derive from the researcher role, the informants or underlying personal difficulties. Knowing the frequency with which these emotional problems happen may help the researcher to get them into perspective. The 'cost of involvement' in research into sensitive topics needs to be discussed more openly.

Completion of the fieldwork and data analysis

Field notes captured my immediate impressions and reactions to the informant and her data. I incorporated new themes into subsequent interviews. After I had listened to the recording of the interview, it was transcribed on to disk. I checked a printed version with the taped interview to correct errors and colloquial and technical terms.

When I had interviewed 23 previous relinquishing mothers and 40 midwives, no new concepts were emerging and the data were complete or 'saturated' (Stern, 1980). Thus, no more interviews were needed. Data analysis began during the fieldwork or data collection. I used comparative analysis (Stern, 1980), in which I compared new with existing data, to determine how they related to each other. Thus, my thoughts were constantly developing and being revised to decide the direction of interviews.

In exploring the experience of relinquishment and the provision of midwifery care, I sought ideas which would highlight the essential aspects of that care. This exploration was completed after each phase of the fieldwork by using analytic description; this involved close scrutiny of the interview transcripts to find new aspects of relinquishment and care. This method of analysis ensured that all of the essential findings had been explained (Macintyre, 1975; Wilson, 1985).

The hard copy was coded using categories which seemed appropriate from my reading of and listening to the interviews. There were about 200 categories for the relinquishing mothers and a similar number for the midwives. Some of the categories were common to both groups, such as the place of care, but there were many which were relevant only to one group of informants, such as mothers giving and midwives learning about grieving. These categories were grouped and reformed into 20 themes, each of which focused on one area. Examination and counting gave me a complete picture, including the importance of all of the aspects (Fielding & Lee, 1991).

Terminology

Anonymity and confidentiality are vital to the informants, so I have used fictitious names. Names ending with 'y' or 'e' (Amy, Betty, Annie, Bessie, etc.) denote midwives, whereas relinquishing mothers have been given names ending with 'a' (Anthea, Barbara, etc.). The names were chosen and given in alphabetical order without regard to the informant's personality.

The opportunities: outstanding research needs

Certain areas relating to perinatal loss still need researching.

Maternity care for the grieving mother

We have considered already in this chapter the dangers of under-researched interventions being applied dogmatically. While Forrest *et al.* (1982) have attempted to look at the effects of interventions to assist grieving, their research design incorporated a 'care package' and the constituent parts were not clearly distinguishable, leaving us wondering which parts were effective. If we are to establish the value of interventions and avoid unjustified dogma, it is necessary for us to learn more about how mothers perceive their care, such as the care of the mother's breasts and whether she lactates (see Chapter 4).

The organisation of the care of the grieving mother deserves attention in that we should find out whether a 'team approach' comprising highly-trained and experienced specialists (Brown, 1992; Dunlop & Hockley, 1990) is more acceptable to the mother than the usual pattern of care (Leon, 1990).

Midwives are accustomed to teaching mothers and others about various aspects of childbearing, but little is known about what is taught to mothers about grief or whether that teaching is effective. It is necessary for us to find out what education is provided and whether the mother and others who are involved perceive it as helpful (see Chapter 4).

The care of the mother in the community

The midwives in my recent study were uniformly convinced of the value of the mother being transferred home promptly:

Hilary   I think that as long as everything's all right she should be able to go home the next day. She should have as short a stay in hospital as possible. In hospital she may be forced to bottle up her emotions. Hospitals are really very busy places, much too busy to allow her to grieve. She should go home to be with her own people and have the chance to be in her own environment.

This widespread assumption contrasts with the observations by Alice Lovell (1984), who identified the mother's perception of being despatched home over-hastily and not for her benefit, but because the staff in the maternity unit had difficulty coping with her presence (see Chapter 4). The decision about the mother's transfer home, particularly who makes it, what influences it and how it relates to education about grieving, deserves closer attention.

For Lovell's sample the return home was not the panacea which mothers and midwives anticipate. The grieving mother found that her friends and family had other preoccupations which limited the support available. If we continue to transfer the grieving mother home quickly, we should at least know the environment to which she is returning and how it compares with the maternity unit. Although they were convinced that the mother would find good support when she returned home, the midwives in my study were less certain of the role of visitors in the maternity unit:

Queeny   The patient is in control of who comes to see her; if she decides she only wants to see her husband today, then that is who she sees. If there is too much of a crowd we may say something.

While this may reflect a common area of conflict, the implications for the grieving mother are particularly serious. We should give attention to the discrepancy between family visiting in the maternity unit needing supervision and assuming the family at home are supportive. Although the midwives, like Queeny, were happy for the mother to decide who visited, I was unable to find out what help, if any, the mother was given in making and implementing this decision.

Mothers' evaluation of home visits by community staff vary hugely (Cooper, 1980; Lovell, 1983; Lovell *et al.*, 1986). The value of this opportunity to provide continuing education and support for the grieving mother should not be underestimated, but existing reports suggest that it is not well-utilised (see Chapter 4). The factors affecting the benefits of these visits need attention.

Staff issues

As recognised in Chapters 9 and 10, staff in the maternity area have difficulty coping with death, and this may affect their care of the mother. Various formats have been and are being used to support staff in coping with death, ranging from 'We're off to the pub' to formal psychologist-led sessions. In view of the serious implications of staff support for all concerned, information is needed on how best it may be organised.

Other issues

The problems of the mother with a *known stillbirth* (see Chapter 3) and who is aware of carrying a dead baby are unique. Her care is influenced by the way in which her grief progresses before her baby is born, but little is currently known about her grieving. To care for this mother optimally we need a more complete picture of how her grief progresses.

The research by Cooper on *parental grief after perinatal death* (1980, see Chapter 2) presents data, such as the parents not perceiving a need to grieve, which conflict with our current view. I have identified certain methodological difficulties which may account for these conflicts, but this study needs replication to provide us with a more complete picture of those for whom we care and their reaction to their loss. Midwives are generally confident to recommend mothers to contact *self-help groups* (see Chapter 11), but the basis of this confidence is unclear and the benefits of these groups deserve research (Watson, 1993).

Mothers belonging to ethnic minority groups are neglected by researchers generally. Research into loss is just one example of the lack of research generally relating to minority groups and demonstrates the ethnocentricity of UK health care (Douglas, 1992). If we are to care appropriately for mothers of different ethnic backgrounds, information about their interpretation of their loss is urgently needed.

Is *maternal death* an appropriate topic in a book about loss in childbearing? My uncertainty relates partly to not having yet been involved in the death of a mother. I find, having discussed this with a small and non-random sample of midwives, that my experience is not unique.

Thoughts about maternal death led my mind first to the unpredictable and seemingly unpreventable 'obstetric accidents' of which all midwives live in fear and which result in the mother dying suddenly in the birthing room or operating theatre. These tragedies are now less likely to involve midwives because a mother whose condition deteriorates is likely to be transferred to a general Intensive Therapy Unit (ITU). It is there that she may die, by which time the ITU nursing staff will be supporting her relatives. Although the midwife in the acute area may be less involved, those who are caring for her baby, in either the postnatal area or the Neonatal Unit (NNU), continue to support the family.

Complacency in western countries may result from maternal death happening only infrequently in developed countries (DoH, 1991), but tragically more often in less-developed countries (Kwast, 1991). However, this is a topic that needs to be researched for two reasons. First, as more mothers are affected by HIV/AIDS, maternal death will become an event which confronts each midwife more frequently (Kell & Barton, 1991). Second, at present we are unable to prepare ourselves for this calamity because the loss of a mother has such dire personal consequences for both family and carers; midwives who have this experience lead me to believe that its impact is earthshattering. For these reasons we need to focus research attention on the psychosocial effects of maternal death and the support which we as carers are able to provide both for the family and for each other when a mother dies.

In contemplating researching this topic, we may be hampered by the lack of relevant literature. While epidemiological and preventative aspects of maternal mortality are well-covered, the care of the mother, her family and the carers are not; exceptionally, a dying mother was discussed in a staff support group (Roch, 1987). The literature from other disciplines may help to illuminate this subject, such as the sudden or unexpected death faced by nurses in the Accident and Emergency department (A&E) (Wright, 1991). Another potentially relevant area is the psychological after-effects of large-scale disasters, such as Hillsborough (Heller, 1993). While the extent of the loss is entirely different, the implications for individual carers may not be (Durham *et al.*, 1985).

The time may be right for us to open this subject up by finding out how those who have encountered maternal death were or were not helped to cope and continue practising (Perry, 1993).

Summary

In this chapter I have considered the significance of research in caring for the grieving mother. I have shown its importance for those who provide care and, indirectly, for the mother herself. After suggesting that research may on occasions be used inappropriately, I have shown how I used a suitably flexible research approach. Finally, I have identified some aspects of loss in childbearing which need research attention.

Chapter 3
Features of Loss in Childbearing

There are certain situations, other than those which come easily to mind, when a mother faces grief. I have already considered the concept of grief in normal, healthy childbearing. I now consider losses which engender profound and enduring grief. In this chapter I focus, first, on those features of loss in childbearing which prolong or inhibit grieving. Second, I contemplate certain examples of loss which present special difficulty.

Features of loss which adversely affect grieving

To examine the unique features, I utilise Davidson's theoretical framework (1977) based on interviews with 15 families with experience of perinatal death. He was able to identify certain aspects of loss which engendered conflict and confusion and impeded healthy grieving.

Confirming perceptually who died

Due to certain unique factors, the fact of the loss of her baby is hard to accept, or may even be resisted, by the mother. Lewis and Bourne (1989) attribute her reaction to the uncertain and bewildering circumstances in which she 'half knows', but has never seen her baby. These writers liken her situation to that following 'missing, presumed dead' verdicts.

Unreality

Ordinarily, when someone dies after the usual life span, those who are left have a variety of tangible and intangible memories. If there is loss in childbearing, these memories do not exist. The mother may have memories of her baby's movements before the birth or she may recall imaginary 'conversations', perhaps willing her baby to quieten down to sleep or pleading with the baby to be born in order to end an interminable pregnancy. The baby's father has even less by which to remember the baby, perhaps only being kicked in the back at night.

The mother's lack of tangible *memories* leaves her wondering 'What am I grieving for?' She may recall a fleeting contact at birth, when she was in a less than ideal state to take everything in. But, as she is mourning a person who is unseen and unknown in the usual way, she finds that the reality of her loss is missing. If the mother's grieving is to proceed she must accept that her baby has been born and has been lost through death or in another way. This loss means inevitably that the baby will not return or be miraculously brought back. Acceptance of the reality of her loss may be assisted by rehearsing the events, either in her mind or with another person.

Just as the lack of memories makes grieving difficult, the lack of a *focus for grief* may also make loss in childbearing unreal. The coffin and funeral have traditionally provided a short-term focus for grief (Mandelbaum, 1959) and the grave has been a source of longer-term reminiscences. But recently ritual has been dispensed with and unmarked graves or incineration have deprived the mother of a focus for her grief (Lewis, 1976; Kowalski, 1980).

The importance of such a focus impressed itself on me in the culture in which I grew up, where mourners return to the house of the dead person and either choose or are given one of their possessions. It may be an item of clothing, a household object or even a houseplant. Although I initially found it macabre, I learned that this object gives the mourner something concrete on which to focus their grief.

Loss of self

The lack of tangible mementoes of a lost baby lends greater significance to those intangible, unseen and usually unspoken fantasies which only the person experiencing them understands. Having been biologically created by the parents, the baby has not only their genetic makeup, but also has invested in it their hopes, dreams and aspirations. Freud (in Rando, 1986a) suggests that parents commit themselves in their baby, in the hope that the baby will develop to gratify their unfulfilled wishes and unachieved plans (Raphael, 1983).

Thus, the baby represents not only a physical, but also a psychological extension of the parents (Rando, 1986). These dreams and aspirations reflect only those characteristics of the mother which she most admires or loves in herself, hence the wish to pass them on. These narcissistic expectations for her child are dashed if the child is lost (Kowalski, 1987; Rando, 1986a), leaving her to grieve for her child and also for some part of herself which may be indistinguishable from her child (Peretz, 1970).

Untimeliness

A mother grieving the loss of her child represents an upset in the correct order of things, and exacerbates the confusion and loss of control which she feels (Kellner & Lake, 1986). These feelings may be aggravated by the mother's perception of herself and her child as a part of the ongoing tapestry of life, which has been brought to an abrupt end (Rando, 1986a). Hence, for parents who regard their child as their 'stake in eternity' a fundamental threat has been posed to the continuity of life, adding a new and frightening significance to their own mortality (Rando, 1986a). Elements of survivor guilt may leave the mother feeling 'It should have been me', further increasing her confusion.

Lack of contact

The mother, like others, may have mistakenly believed that love only develops when the baby is seen and known (Bowlby, 1969). Because they assume that little contact means no affection, it may be thought that no loving mother–child relationship exists. In contrast to her expectations, the mother may be alarmed by the strength of her emotions making her fear that she is 'going crazy' (Borg & Lasker, 1982). Hence, because she is not regarded as a 'proper' mother, both the mother and those nearby have difficulty accepting the mother's profound and enduring grief. This leads to those near her denigrating her grief, and encouraging her to 'pull herself together'.

Getting emotional support

The non-involvement in childbearing of those who ordinarily give support may limit the help available in the event of loss.

Intimacy of loss

Because, in childbearing, the number of people who have any direct or intimate contact with the baby is unlikely to be more than two, there is little scope for community support. As mentioned already, those not intimately involved have difficulty comprehending the significance of the loss, causing them to make unintentionally hurtful 'Have another'-type comments (Kellner & Lake, 1986).

This difficulty has led to grieving parents being regarded as having no right to grieve; they become the 'illegitimate mourners' (Nichols, 1984). Emotional support is soon withdrawn from those perceived as being undeserving of it. Those who are grieving, quickly realise the futility of seeking help and, so, conceal their emotions, creating a 'conspiracy of silence' and worsening feelings of the birth having been a 'non-event' (Helmrath & Steinitz, 1978; Kowalski, 1983; Kellner & Lake, 1986).

Complexity of emotional processes

While I have shown that the *depth* of grief experienced at this time may be hard for both the mother and those near to her to understand, thus jeopardising her support, the complexity of her emotions may be similarly incomprehensible.

The difficulty is summarised by Hutchins (1986) as saying 'hello and goodbye' simultaneously. During pregnancy, the focus is to prepare a suitable physical and emotional environment in which the new arrival may be nurtured. As the pregnancy advances the momentum of preparations increases, so that completing the necessary emotional 'about-turn', in the event of loss, is a major problem. In Chapter 12 I discuss the problems women encounter if they conceive while mourning. The problems of the new mother mourning her baby are marginally less, as she must finish her optimistic preparations while simultaneously grieving the loss of the mother–child relationship (Lewis & Bourne, 1989).

Relative youth of parents
A women in her childbearing years is relatively young and unlikely to be acquainted with grief (Borg & Lasker, 1982). She will not, therefore, have had opportunities to develop coping strategies to help her through this experience of loss. Thus, her grief becomes a crisis for which, by definition, any previous coping strategies are inappropriate (Caplan, 1961). The ineffective coping strategies utilised by younger bereaved parents are anger and outrage (Cooper, 1980). While their older equivalents also grieve angrily, their anger is underpinned by fear of remaining childless as the mother's biological clock ticks inexorably away.

Appropriate emotional support
While emotional support may be forthcoming, the mother has difficulty identifying who is prepared to offer her sufficiently intensive and enduring support. I discuss family and carers in Chapter 6 and 9 respectively.

Comparing her feelings with those of others

The non-comprehension of the mother's grief by those from whom she ordinarily takes her behavioural cues leaves her feeling unsupported.

Meaning of the pregnancy
The mother's perception of poor support causes her to feel alone and isolated in her grief. One of the factors which aggravates her loneliness is the uniqueness of the meaning which she attaches to her pregnancy (Rando, 1986a). This is because, as mentioned already, when a child is conceived a variety of unique hopes, expectations and aspirations develop in those who are involved (Kowalski, 1987; Rando, 1986a). If a baby is lost, these dreams are also lost and in the same way as the dreams were unique, so is the grief following their loss, leaving the mother isolated (Lewis & Bourne, 1989; Rando, 1986a).

Contrasting her own earlier feelings

The media emphasise the ease and normality of conception, pregnancy and childbearing. This emphasis, together with the widespread secrecy surrounding loss in childbearing, successfully shields us from the relatively infrequent, tragic outcomes (Lewis, 1976; Borg & Lasker, 1982). So, if problems happen, events are shockingly different from expectations; the mother's confidence is shaken and her self-esteem plummets.

Similar assumptions which we make about the ease of childbearing result in an overwhelming focus on control, or prevention, of fertility by contraception. When faced with involuntary infertility, the reality is a shocking contrast to our usual assumptions. The contrast between expectations and reality applies at a fundamental level to all aspects of 'reproductive failure'. Until problems are encountered, fertility is little more than an occasionally inconvenient, basic human function. But when we find that the desired level of fertility is beyond our grasp, our human integrity is threatened (Quirk, 1979; Rando, 1986a).

Examples of loss in childbearing

In addition to these issues which apply generally, each of the more profound forms of loss carry unique features, some of which have been researched.

Stillbirth

Stillbirth, as I have suggested already and as emerges in the research by Cooper (1980) on parental reactions to stillbirth, is a topic which is not discussed socially despite families having knowledge or experience of it. I realised this when I first entered midwifery and mothers told me that the shop always kept the new pram until after the birth 'in case anything happened'. The possibility of stillbirth was recognised implicitly, together with an element of magical thinking to avoid tempting fate.

The research which has been done on this subject has focused on reactions to stillbirth, and care *after* the birth to help cope with those reactions. Probably for this reason, little attention has been given to the two significantly different forms of stillbirth, known and unexpected, and their emotional implications.

Known stillbirth

Sometimes known as intra-uterine death (IUD), maceration may happen, depending on the length of time between the baby's death and birth.

The mother's grieving may be affected by how long she is aware of carrying her dead baby within her. Jolly (1987) suggests that the mother would be the first to note the cessation of fetal movements and realise its significance, leading us to wonder whether this would assist grieving. While Jolly considers that grieving begins only when the baby separates from the mother at birth, Hutchins (1986) maintains that the mother may, beneficially, begin grieving antenatally; she may at least experience shock and denial to begin her grieving prior to the birth or, alternatively, she may begin anticipatory grieving (see Chapter 8).

We need authoritative research evidence about whether and how this woman's grief develops if we are to offer her the most appropriate care.

When carrying a dead baby, the feeling of empty stillness which the mother senses within her symbolises the end of her relationship with her baby (Kellner & Lake, 1986). No longer does her body house a person who is going to provide her with gratification, but she now despises parts of her body that once provided recognition and pleasure.

I will never forget my sense of repugnance when, as a nursing student, I learned that a mother with a known stillbirth was coming into the labour ward for a third attempt to induce labour. I soon realised that her feelings of horror could only be worse than mine, probably akin to the perception of being a 'living coffin' (Jolly, 1987). Profound disturbances in a mother's body image feature uncleanness, which may be associated with her sense of horror at retaining her dead baby (Grubb 1976; Kish 1978).

Forrest (1983) describes the fantasies of such mothers in her sample as being 'unpleasant'. When they voiced concerns about how their babies were physically changing, they were accused of being 'morbid' or 'ghoulish'. Probably unjustifiably, Hutchins blames such anxieties on the mother's inexperience with dead beings.

Because of the physical changes in the baby, the likely emotional reaction and the risk of the mother developing a clotting disorder, *induction of labour* is usually recommended (Llewellyn-Jones, 1990). Traditionally, this induction has been begun speedily, although the labour tends to be protracted; but now there is greater flexibility about whether the mother or professionals decide whether and when the induction happens. Dyer (1992) encourages waiting 'a day or two' for induction after learning of her loss, for the mother to reorientate herself.

Assuming that she will see her baby, the changes in the baby's body may affect the mother's decision about when to have labour induced (Hutchins, 1986). Delaying the induction may signify continuing denial, although this need not indicate an early induction. The mother deciding the timing of the induction may be one way for her to assume control of an otherwise uncontrollable situation (see below, Kellner & Lake, 1986). Midwives in my recent study encouraged this mother's control (Mander, 1992d):

Ottily   [Induction] is an obstetrician's decision though, but I think that they move too fast sometimes and that may not be good for the woman, it may not be healthy for her. It seems to be a case of 'get it over and done with'. I think that this may be for the benefit of the staff – for us. One woman was asked to come in that same afternoon. She didn't come in and she actually turned up three days later. We had been in touch with her GP to check that there were no real problems and it seemed to be alright. She waited until she felt that she was ready. But the labour is usually induced as soon as the diagnosis of fetal death has been made. This is probably blocking the realisation of the death. When it is being explained to the woman she would probably be told about the medical risks such as DIC [Disseminated Intravascular Coagulation] and coagulation problems.

If the woman is still protecting herself from the unacceptable news by *denial*, the staff may be unable to convince her of the reality of her baby's death. I learned this when I was a new midwife in an antenatal ward and a mother with hypertension was admitted near term. Our observations indicated that her baby was dead, but she insisted that this was not so because her baby was still moving. Despite being gently informed of the situation, her denial persisted. Days later, she agreed to have labour induced because her baby was due and her blood pressure remained high. She was inconsolable when her daughter was stillborn. Hutchins (1986) and Cooper (1980) discuss the ways in which denial may be used and the effect that this may have on others, such as family. It is not, however, only mothers who use denial as protection; a midwife informant recounted her experience of known stillbirth:

Annie   There is a moment at the birth when everyone who is present, the parents and the staff, see that the baby has been born and hope against hope that the baby is going to cry. I know that it's quite illogical, but you still hope. And it is not until that moment when we all realise that the baby really is dead, that we all finally realise it is so.

Unexpected stillbirth

The baby may die unexpectedly in labour or at birth, resulting in what may be known as a fresh stillbirth. This death has all the characteristics of sudden death (Hutchins, 1986), with the parents experiencing 'numbing shock and paralysing fear, with little time for mythical bargaining'. This form of stillbirth may only be recognised when we are unable to resuscitate a previously healthy baby whose condition at birth was poor. Ethical questions arise when deciding how long to continue resuscitation attempts.

The unexpectedness of this form of loss presents a major challenge to the staff as well as the mother. They may question the reliability of their own observations which led to confidence in the baby's condition. They may find that those aspects of care which are ordinarily second nature, such as communication and information-giving, become unbearably difficult. In my experience, the mother's needs for information and support may be overlooked while staff continue resuscitation attempts and face the prospect of a healthy fetus becoming a stillbirth.

Reactions after the birth

The depths of mothers' reactions to stillbirth have been shown in two rather different studies. Wolff *et al.* (1970) described the allocation of blame and effect on future childbearing, whereas Cullberg (1971) researched the mothers' psychological distress.

Wolff and others followed up a group of 50 relatively young mothers for up to three years. Half of the group attempted to find solace in a 'replacement child' (see Chapter 12), whereas the remainder were so keen to avoid another pregnancy that a large proportion were sterilised. Blame was attributed approximately equally to the mother, the father, fate or God. These researchers, unlike Cullberg, identified no evidence of psychiatric illness.

The sample and time scale in Cullberg's study were similar to Wolff's, but one-third of the mothers reported sufficiently severe symptoms to justify a diagnosis of psychiatric illness. The level of detail provided by Cullberg indicates that the measurements were reliable, whereas in Wolff this is less clear, indicating that the more serious outcome may be accurate.

Research

While the research by Wolff *et al.* (1970) and by Cullberg (1971) helps to illuminate the experience of mothers of stillborn babies, the age of these studies and their North American and Northern European origins make it necessary to question their relevance in this rapidly changing area.

In a more recent UK study of 17 couples, Cooper (1980) drew on her social work background and highlighted the perception of poor communication between health professionals and mothers and also the lack of communication between the parents. These perceptions were reflected in the lack of warmth and humanity encountered by the mothers in hospital as shown by comments such as:

'I felt like a piece of meat – no longer human'.
'Once you're in [hospital] you don't belong to yourself any more.'

The mothers in this sample did not see their babies and Cooper questions the terms in which the offer to see the baby was couched. The decision not to see the baby may have been influenced by the fathers in that, despite denial being common, they were anxious that contact might impair the mother's self-control.

The prevalent emotional response among these parents was found to be anger; this more masculine response reflects the powerful male orientation of Cooper's report, an example being the ostracism reported by the husbands at work and the need for the woman to be protected, that is isolated, from family for about a week. The couples in this study perceived stillbirth as a threat to their marriage, status and role and as a medical accident involving the failure of a physiological process, but not as a bereavement requiring mourning.

Although Cooper illuminates the responses of a certain group of people at a certain time, the research needs to be replicated to probe in greater depth reactions to health care and other emotional aspects of stillbirth. Cooper does not indicate whether each couple was interviewed together; individual interviews might present a more accurate picture of the mother's feelings. The need for more authoritative research in this area has been identified elsewhere (Adams & Prince, 1991), but the research must advance our knowledge and practice based on existing work, such as Cooper's, rather than disregarding it.

Accidental loss in early pregnancy: miscarriage

A pregnancy may be accidentally lost before becoming viable in any of a number of ways including spontaneous abortion and ectopic pregnancy. Although the circumstances of the loss differ markedly, I use the word 'miscarriage' to include these various forms of loss.

A common event

Although the loss of 'biological' pregnancies may be much higher (Oakley *et al.*, 1990), clinically-recognised miscarriages are estimated to occur in up to 31% of all pregnancies (Bansen & Stevens, 1992). The frequency of miscarriage leads some to regard it as a normal event (Roberts, 1989). This information may be used to 'comfort' the woman who has experienced a miscarriage, by telling her that it is 'nature's way' of preventing the birth of a baby with disabilities (Iles, 1989). Such denigration of the experience may eventually lead to the baby being described as products of conception (POC) (Wesson, 1989).

Grieving miscarriage

Our traditional disregard of miscarriage may be attributable to the following:

(1) the non-visibility and resulting non-recognition of the pregnancy (Bansen & Stevens, 1992)
(2) the assumption in the past that 'quickening' is highly significant in the development of both the fetus and the mother–baby relationship, rendering earlier loss less meaningful

(3) our limited knowledge of the emotional processes of early pregnancy, which may include the assumption that shorter gestation
carries less emotional investment.

There is evidence to suggest that the emotional changes which assist the
adjustment to parenthood may begin prior to conception (Rubin, 1967)
and in a large and authoritative study it was found that there are no
significant differences between the grief responses of women losing
their babies through miscarriage, stillbirth or neonatal death (Peppers &
Knapp, 1980). Assumption of 'no grief' following miscarriage, may be
little more than an admission of ignorance, because no-one follows-up
this mother to find out how she does or does not recover (Iles, 1989). It
may be that by dismissing this mother's emotional response to
miscarriage, we may be denying her the opportunity to grieve healthily.
   Research into grief following miscarriage has focused on the
psychiatric sequelae. An important example is a North American study
(Cain *et al.*, 1964) which, unfortunately, utilised a sample of psychiatric
patients. These researchers identified the significant feelings of grief,
guilt, failure, fear for future childbearing and anger at the father and the
gynaecologist. In a better-designed study (Leppert & Pahlka, 1984),
grief following miscarriage was shown to be as intense as grief for other
perinatal loss, as Peppers and Knapp found, and the pattern was similar
to grieving adult loss. Using telephone interviews, the researchers found
that grief lasted for between three and four months before resolution
began.
   The value of earlier work to measure the emotional consequences of
miscarriage has been questioned on the grounds of non-use of a
standardised assessment (Friedman & Gath, 1989). These researchers
used well-validated depression scales and the Present State Examination
(PSE) to assess the mental state of 67 women four weeks after
miscarriage. A semi-structured interview preceded a psychiatric
assessment. The PSE showed that 32 mothers (48%) were psychiatric
'cases', a rate four times higher than women generally. The psychiatric
condition was invariably of a depressive nature and correlated with
previous miscarriage rather than childlessness. Many of the mothers
showed features typical of grief and three had attempted self-harm.

The experience of miscarriage
In view of the tendency, mentioned already, to denigrate the
significance of miscarriage, Bansen and Stevens (1992) undertook a
qualitative study to describe the experience of early miscarriage. The
sample of 10 mothers who had miscarried two to five months earlier
was gathered through referrals and informal networking. The mothers
had all lost a first desired pregnancy.
   These researchers found profound guilt, anger at their bodies and fear

for future childbearing. Most significantly, this study showed that miscarriage is not necessarily the insignificant menstruation-like event which is sometimes thought (Roberts, 1989), as several mothers focused on the pain and heavy bleeding which were severe enough to engender fear of dying.

The mothers' grief was long-lasting; resolution of their grief may have been impeded by the sudden onset of their miscarriage, precluding any opportunities for anticipatory grieving. Social support was unforthcoming, which was compounded by unhelpful comments denigrating the loss.

Regarding her future, each mother was consoled by having conceived and the fact of her pregnancy convinced her that she would be able to conceive again. The miscarriage shattered the mothers' complacency about their fertility, which changed their outlook for future childbearing by making them feel vulnerable.

Ritual and recognition

The absence of ritual for mourning miscarriage has been observed (Leppert & Pahlka, 1984); although parents may resent the need to register a stillborn baby (Cooper, 1980), it constitutes a recognition of their loss. In the UK, registration of miscarriage is not required, neither is burial or other ritual, although memorial services are increasingly available (Roberts, 1989).

Termination of pregnancy for fetal abnormality

UK legislation (1967) states that termination of pregnancy (TOP) is not illegal in certain circumstances; these include 'social' reasons as well as situations in which there is 'a substantial risk that if the child was born it would suffer from such physical or mental abnormalities as to be seriously handicapped'. When undertaken for the latter reason TOP may be known as termination for fetal abnormality.

Since this legislation was enacted there has been a plethora of research on the emotional outcomes of 'social' TOP. The lobby seeking to reverse or at least amend the legislation has been influential in initiating some of this research. Whether the general finding of limited adverse emotional sequelae occurring after 'social' TOP applies to termination for fetal abnormality must be addressed. The situation is crucially different because termination for fetal abnormality is undertaken when the pregnancy, though possibly unplanned, has continued until the prenatal diagnosis procedures are undertaken, suggesting that it is wanted (Laurence, 1989; Richards, 1989).

Cultural implications

TOP is contentious and raises ethical issues. In some countries legislation is still under debate. This ongoing debate must affect our use of literature from countries such as the USA. We should also bear in mind the effects of certain religious groups whose attitudes to TOP may be carried over into the area of termination for fetal abnormality (Kenyon, 1988).

Frequency
The proportion of TOPs carried out because of the risk of fetal abnormality is a fairly constant 1–2% (Iles, 1989; Richards, 1989). The proportion of late TOPs (after 20 weeks) undertaken for fetal abnormality is considerably larger at over 17%.

Decision-making
The series of decisions which may end with the mother grieving the loss of her baby through termination for fetal abnormality will have begun much earlier, possibly before she ever contemplated pregnancy. Whether she is able to take advantage of prenatal diagnosis depends on high-level policy decisions about whether they are to be available in her locality and whether she meets the criteria, such as a lower age limit for amniocentesis (Reid, 1990).

The reasons for women deciding to accept prenatal diagnosis were explored in a study by Farrant (1985), which illuminated the conflicting views held by mothers and their medical advisers. Farrant found that mothers seek the 'all-clear' to allow their pregnancies to continue confidently, while the priority for obstetricians is the diagnosis and abortion of affected fetuses.

The decisions open to mothers may be limited by obstetricians' concern about 'wasting' resources. Some may require a commitment that, should a positive diagnosis be made, the mother will go through with termination for fetal abnormality (Richards, 1989:177; Borg & Lasker, 1982). While decisions are assumed to be made on the basis of complete information, this may not always be forthcoming. Farrant's examples include the priority obstetricians give to abnormal results and the general failure to inform of normal results, expecting mothers to conclude that no news is good news.

Hypothetical decisions were sought by Green *et al.* (1993) in their study of attitudes to prenatal diagnosis and termination for fetal abnormality in 1824 pregnant women. These researchers showed that women's unwillingness to contemplate termination for fetal abnormality did not prevent them from accepting prenatal diagnosis, and they suggest that this apparent contradiction may be explained in three ways:

(1) Women's lack of understanding of the 'PND Package' may prevent them from making the connection between prenatal diagnosis and termination for fetal abnormality. Prenatal diagnosis may be viewed

as merely hurdles to be overcome to ensure a healthy baby, possibly regardless of test results. There may be an element of magical thinking in this attitude (see below).
(2) Being informed about the baby's condition may help a woman to prepare for the birth of an affected baby.
(3) In endorsement of Farrant's observation, first and foremost mothers seek reassurance, rendering attitudes to termination for fetal abnormality of little consequence.

The 'enormous' pressures applied to mothers to go through with termination for fetal abnormality have been identified by Rothman (1990); in North America these include:

(1) Financial pressure, by the provision of less state support to people with disabilities.
(2) Pressure in individual women who may feel guilty at choosing to give birth to individuals who are treated so badly.
(3) Social pressure, deriving more and more from the view that disability is the direct responsibility of the mother and less as divine or any other intervention.

These pressures may result in the situation identified in the study by Donnai *et al.* (1981) of the grief reactions of 12 mothers who had undergone termination for fetal abnormality. Guilt did not feature among this sample because such a termination was thought appropriate. The exception was one mother who was still 'very distressed' a year after her termination because she thought that the pregnancy should have continued despite fetal abnormality.

Giving bad news
For a small proportion of the mothers accepting prenatal diagnosis it will be necessary for them to be given bad news in clinical situations such as the ultrasound department. Statham and Dimavicius (1992) discuss how this painful situation may best be handled, reminding us of parents' sensitivity to anything being 'not quite right'. The authors discuss the problem of the ultrasound technician who is competent to identify a problem but lacks authority to explain it to the parents. The authors suggest how to handle the seemingly interminable wait to be 'told officially' without aggravating the distress of the parents or those waiting their turn. Jargon is ruled out and the parents viewing the screen to see the problem is recommended to provide maximum information.

The effect on the developing emotional relationship
Prenatal diagnosis may affect the development of the mother's love for her baby by resetting her emotional clock in several ways. The mother

may not permit herself to love her baby until she has the 'all-clear'. The 'tentative pregnancy' (Rothman, 1986) puts the emotional relationship 'on hold' pending the results.

The emotional relationship may be facilitated by seeing the baby on ultrasound scan (Lumley, 1980; Richards, 1989). Richards recounts how, unfortunately, the magical significance of this experience may be lost on the ultrasound technician.

Once the mother has successfully negotiated the hurdles of prenatal diagnosis, her 'tentative' stance is shed as she swings into pregnancy mode, allowing herself to suddenly bloom (Richards, 1989). The celebration of a normal result may anticipate, or even supplant, the celebration of the birth.

I have already referred to mothers' limited understanding of prenatal diagnosis and have used the term 'all-clear' to describe mothers' interpretation of the results because of the not uncommon assumption that because prenatal diagnosis has revealed no problems the baby must be perfect (Reid, 1990:304; Richards, 1989). Perhaps the mother, having convinced herself of normality, may react inappropriately badly to a more minor problem, such as an extra digit.

Psychological sequelae

Although some may assume that the woman's only reaction after termination for fetal abnormality is one of relief at having avoided the birth of a baby with a handicap (Iles, 1989), the reality is less straightforward. As with other situations, we assume that because we don't see the problems, they don't exist. Iles (1989) suggests six reasons why termination for fetal abnormality is associated with emotions other than relief:

(1) These are wanted pregnancies, as mentioned already.
(2) Because termination for fetal abnormality is undertaken later, the demise of the pregnancy will be obvious to those around, requiring explanations and risking criticism (Borg & Lasker, 1982). Additionally, 'labour' is a longer and more distressing event.
(3) Handicaps not incompatible with life produce guilt in the mother for not keeping and coping with the child (Harris, 1986).
(4) The risk of recurrence may threaten future childbearing.
(5) In older mothers the chances of successful childbearing may be diminishing.
(6) The abnormality in the fetus, conceived by the parents, engenders guilt and lowered self-esteem at the failure of a normal process. Guilt is doubled, on the grounds of failed reproduction *and* deciding on termination for fetal abnormality (Raphael-Leff, 1991; Blumberg *et al.*, 1975; Harris, 1986).

The difficulty of the mother's grieving following this type of termination is attributed to the baby being unseen, the lack of a grave, and trivialisation of the mother's loss (Lloyd & Laurence, 1985; Iles, 1989). This difficulty was confirmed in a later retrospective study of 48 women following termination for fetal abnormality, in which 36 mothers (75%) experienced an acute grief reaction (Laurence, 1989). The reactions were sufficiently severe for 21% of the mothers to need psychiatric help. These highly significant figures may be compared with the incidence of grief following TOP for 'social' reasons, when only 5% of mothers are affected. Laurence found that previous experience of perinatal loss was associated with easier and quicker resolution of grief, although eight of the ten mothers who had a 'risk factor' still experienced an acute grief reaction. These mothers felt that the 'voluntariness' of their decision to have a termination for fetal abnormality, far from easing their grief, had aggravated it.

Because of the limitations of previous studies on emotional reactions following termination for fetal abnormality, Iles' prospective study used standardised measures as well as semi-structured interviews (1989). Seventy-one mothers were interviewed on three occasions in the year following such termination. A large proportion (39%) of the mothers were identified as psychiatric 'cases' using PSE. Iles indicates that psychiatric problems fell to general population levels by the time of the second interview at six months, although less serious symptoms of anxiety and depression may persist. Iles relates these symptoms to unresolved guilt and anxiety about future childbearing. The psychiatric outcome is worse if the abnormality was non life-threatening or if the termination for fetal abnormality was later.

Knowledge and its use

Richards (1989) argues that in this context as in others, our knowledge is outstripping our ability to use it safely. Although research demonstrates the problems which women may encounter following termination for fetal abnormality, it remains to be seen whether our care is able to reduce these problems.

Newborns with handicaps

The concerns commonly experienced by the pregnant mother may not prepare her for the reality of her baby being born with an unexpected handicap (Niven, 1992). The maternity staff need to understand the extent of the adjustments which are required of her if she is to love and care for her baby. Some may think that because of prenatal diagnosis, no babies are born with unexpected disabilities. But, perhaps because of the machinery being used, the human being using it or the mother not availing herself of prenatal diagnosis, babies may still be born with unexpected handicaps (Chitty *et al.*, 1991).

Terminology and definition

The terminology used to describe a newborn baby with handicaps varies hugely. While avoiding any suggestion that a baby with a handicap is deficient, it is essential to emphasise their difference from other babies and from the baby which had been expected. For this reason and recognising its limitations I, like Niven, use the terminology which parents are likely to understand and use.

In thinking about handicap I include a wide range of problems which become apparent neonatally. They may be more or less serious and have a similarly wide variety of implications for the baby and the family. Although the mother's reaction is likely to follow a certain pattern, the depth and duration of her response will vary according to the meaning she attributes to this baby and to the handicap. I look at the situation when the baby's survival is uncertain in Chapter 8.

Grieving

The response to handicap is essentially similar to the grief reaction which we encounter in other situations (Irvin *et al.*, 1982). This mother needs to grieve the loss of the perfect baby about whom she had fantasised and end that relationship (Solnit & Stark, 1961). Over-powering emotional demands are placed on her by the need, at the same time, to come to accept and grow to love her real baby with the handicap (Roberts, 1977). She may develop feelings of unreality due to uncertainty of who the baby is; whether the baby being mourned is perfect or the real baby who needs loving care and attention.

Denial may feature prominently in this mother's grief, and may be temporarily helpful, as in a mother I cared for whose baby showed features of Down's syndrome. When informed of the likely diagnosis, she retorted that 'He looks just like his dad'. It was interesting to find that her observation was correct, but investigations confirmed the diagnosis, by which time she was coming to know and love her son.

Another significant feature of this mother's grief is her occasional feeling that her child might be better off dead (Lewis & Bourne, 1989). Such thoughts are alarming. They aggravate the feelings of guilt which grief invariably carries with it and may give rise to clinical depression. Roberts recommends that parents should be warned that these guilt-provoking thoughts will emerge, in the hope that the mother will not be too frightened by her own feelings.

Because of her feeling that grief is inappropriate, the mother may never complete her grieving. Her relationship with her real baby is, therefore, unable to become established and her grief may reappear unpredictably with future losses (see Chapter 6).

Breaking the news

The circumstances in which the parents learn of their child's handicap will vary according to its nature, but the method of being told is viewed critically. Dissatisfaction with the way the information was given among parents of babies with Down's syndrome is clear (Cunningham *et al.*, 1984). This study also shows that this is not simply a case of 'shooting the messenger'.

Looking to the future
Because a baby is perceived as comprising the characteristics which the mother values most highly in herself (see above), the birth of a baby with a handicap represents an additional narcissistic insult to her self-esteem (Leon, 1990). This feeling may be aggravated by the child being an ever-present reminder of both the parents' loss of their perfect baby and their own failure (Raphael-Leff, 1991).

The parents' feelings of guilt and the likelihood of recrimination and blame within the relationship emerged in my recent study. A midwife recalled a mother who had just relinquished her Down's syndrome baby for adoption at the insistence of her husband:

> *Marie* ... maybe she was frightened to come and see the baby in case she did form an attachment to the baby and took it home and it would end her marriage. If, you know, at the end of the day, she takes that baby home she might end up losing her husband. She's left with one child, an abnormal handicapped child, to cope with as well, and no husband.

Relinquishment

Although it is widely accepted (Roll *et al.*, 1986; Sorosky *et al.*, 1984) that grieving following relinquishment has many features in common with grieving loss through death, there are certain crucial differences. The data from my recent study suggest that, as in any grief, there is a capacity for deviation from the general pattern. Certain deviations which may impede grieving appeared regularly among the mothers I interviewed, leading to the conclusion that there is scope for intervention to benefit the mother who relinquishes her baby.

Delay in grieving
Bowlby (1980) includes delayed grieving as a pathological state and associates it with an apparently voluntary avoidance of the pain of loss. For a small number of the relinquishing mothers the voluntariness was clear:

> *Iona*   OK, so I grieved when I was in hospital. I cried nearly all week ... But I think you can't just shut off something like that completely, which is what I tried to do.

The extent to which the delayed grieving experienced by relinquishing mothers is voluntary must be questioned, as many appear to have had some external pressure applied to 'conform' in the interests of secrecy and to benefit the family:

Barbara   Because I had had to go from the hospital home, the circumstances of my dad's mother staying, having to pretend that nothing had happened and in effect not being allowed to mourn . . . I hadn't been allowed to do any of this.

Relinquishment usually happens while the woman is relatively young, so that her life soon becomes filled with events that may impede her grieving. These events may involve family responsibilities:

Hilda   It's getting worse now because I had the boys to think of, so that kept it in the background. Now the boys are grown up, I think more now. I was busy with them and its hurting worse now.

Work-related factors also serve to impede grieving:

Nadia   I find that the sorrow deepens, and that the guilt is always present. The years after I placed him for adoption were busy years for me and my husband. I was having the children and he was building up the business. This prevented me from grieving properly for the loss of my baby.

Occasionally, work was regarded by the mother, with help from those near her, as therapeutic in dealing with overt grief. Some, like Jessica, soon realised that the therapy she had been recommended was merely papering over the cracks:

Jessica   I had no outlet and so there are lots of feelings which have never been let out. The main thing was to get back to work.

It is clear that for the relinquishing mother, her grieving is suspended while she, with the connivance of others, gets on with her life. The reactivation of her grief when her life is less busy is a shock, although there is another factor, the inability to let go (see below), which exacerbates the grief when it does manifest itself:

Barbara   I had to go for counselling at the — [Psychiatric] Hospital. I didn't have to go back because it had all come out. Hours of crying turned out to be what I hadn't been allowed to do then. I'm sure if I hadn't seen that TV programme it would still be inside and something somewhere along the line would have unlocked it, you know? So I think a lot of feelings then weren't allowed to come out – at the time or after – perhaps at the time of the birth.

Inability to share grief
In emphasising the 'shared' nature of grief, Clark (1991) raises the

inevitability of death for all of us and thus the community experience in which the bereaved person is nurtured and sustained by those around. It may be that relinquishment is perceived as a deviant form of behaviour in a society, such as the UK, where the prevailing pattern is for every mother to care for her own baby. This perception of being deviant and being stigmatised, described by Lena as 'shame', was strongly felt by some mothers:

Ursula I think that a hospital is there to give care to people, not a courtroom where you are judged for what you have or have not done. This midwife did this, because when she read my notes her attitude to me changed. She had been kind and welcoming when I came into the labour ward, but after she read them she was chilly. I asked her 'Have you read my notes now?' She said 'Yes'.

This perception was also reported by some midwives:

Gay I think secrecy's quite important for certain people, yes . . . because for some people unmarried mothers are still, especially out in the country, it seems to be very much frowned upon. Yeah. I don't really think we are as permissive as all that. I think people like to think we are, but I don't think we are.

Jones (1989) discusses grief in the context of another group, gay men, who may be stigmatised or regarded as deviant, though he prefers to discuss the 'absence of recognition' of their relationship. Because the relationship is not sanctioned by society the bereaved partner may not be offered the support usually available to the bereaved person and, Jones maintains, their grief work may be inhibited. If the relationship of the relinquishing mother with her baby is similarly unrecognised, she may find herself not only being isolated from this essential community support, but possibly additionally being stigmatised for her deviant behaviour in parting from her baby. This silent isolation was clear:

Kara I found it really hard to adjust myself back into a normal [lifestyle] . . . it was like mourning a bereavement. It is like somebody's died but when somebody dies it is different because it is talked about.

To Clark (1991) the significance of the funeral is fundamental: 'While we have been robbed of relatedness and are threatened with broken-ness, through coming together to remember and to honour the person who has died, we affirm the vitality of our bonds with others.'

Although a funeral is accepted and expected if a baby dies perinatally (Borg & Lasker, 1982), the mother who relinquishes has no equivalent rite of passage:

Debra   On the day when I gave her up I dressed her ready for the adoptive
parents. My parents and me were sitting in a bare room and I had planned
what I would do when I handed her over, adjusting her shawl and everything. Then the social worker came and said 'I'll take your baby now' and
she did. I was unable to do any of the things I'd planned – no ceremony, no
kiss or anything. It's the hardest thing I've ever done, I'll never get over it.
(*Tears*).

A mother who relinquished her baby more recently was able to arrange
the ceremony which she wanted:

Olivia   My parents are Mormons and . . . I arranged for our church leader to
come in and bless her. I felt that this was appropriate. We had to go into the
utility room to do it. My flatmate was there and her boyfriend and my
younger brother. It was not really a goodbye ceremony it was more a way of
recognising her as my child that is a part of me to go to Christian parents.
The blessing was my way of establishing the baby's rights as an individual, a
way of recognising the break from being mine. The blessing was the right
thing to do . . .

Letting go
Clark (1991) suggests that even in normal, healthy grieving it may
never actually be possible to 'let go' of the one who dies. He
suggests that the terms 'integration' or 'consolidation' may better
describe the final stage of the grieving process. If this is so, it raises
the question of whether there is any possibility of the relinquishing
mother *ever* completing this stage of grieving in view of her profound awareness of the possibility of the physical reappearance of
the relinquished one. The work of Bouchier *et al*., (1991) establishes
the widespread prevalence of the desire to resume contact with the
one who was relinquished and touches on the effect of this desire on
the mother's grieving. The mothers in the present study were all
aware of the possibility of future contact:

Jessica   I often think about the possibility of my child trying to trace me and
make contact . . .
Rosa   I'd be [delighted] if he would turn up on the doorstep.

It is clearly apparent that for the mother who relinquished her baby, the
possibility, even hope, of future contact is genuine. Some mothers
demonstrated a real awareness that the lack of a conclusion to the
relationship impedes complete grieving:

Lena   But sometimes I think when you're young and you have them
adopted it's like a death – its a bereavement when you lose it, y'know.
But if you lose somebody through death, you know that that's them
gone. When you give up your baby you know that it is somewhere else.

Sometimes I think I wish she had died then I would know that I might see her again [after death].

These comments would appear to reinforce the observation by Bouchier *et al.* (1991): 'The balance between loss and hope is a difficult one for all human beings to maintain.'

Non-completion of grieving
Despite definite similarities between relinquishment and loss through death, which indicate that relinquishment is a form of bereavement, lack of any conclusion impedes the resolution of grief due to relinquishment.

Infertility

Grieving a child may seem inappropriate in a couple who have not even been able to conceive. Such uncomprehending attitudes aggravate the feelings of the infertile couple. In this section I consider whether grief is relevant in this context and, if so, the factors which may affect the couple's grief.

Definition and incidence
When we discuss 'infertility' we tend to assume the 'involuntary' prefix; I am discussing involuntary childlessness, rather than voluntary infertility which results in the couple being 'child-free' (Campbell, 1985). Although occasionally defined as the inability to have the number of children which they desire, infertility is ordinarily defined in terms of the duration of unprotected sexual intercourse without conception, usually one year, but when the couple seeks help will vary according to factors such as their age, lifestyle and cultural background.

The incidence of infertility varies according to the criteria which are used to define it, but the usual estimate is that about 15% of couples are childless (Menning, 1982). The majority of couples who consider themselves infertile have not had *any* children, but over 33% of couples who are investigated for infertility are having difficulty conceiving a subsequent child (Dor *et al.*, 1977).

Responses
Frank (1984) describes the grief of the infertile couple as relating to an abstract or potential loss rather than the tangible loss which has featured to a greater or lesser extent in the other forms of loss which I have considered. Theirs is not the actual but the potential loss of their child, of their childbearing experience and of being a parent. They grieve not only their lack of a child, but also their loss of genetic continuity and their loss of fertility (Menning, 1982). The fact that this is a totally abstract

loss does not facilitate the couple's grieving and may make it more difficult (Frank, 1984).

Although this couple's grief has much in common with the grief which we know happens in many settings, it also has certain unique features. First, the realisation of an infertility problem dawns on the couple as a total surprise (Menning, 1982). We are accustomed to assuming that we are fertile and to taking the appropriate action to control, or rather limit, it. This assumption continues into the area of childbearing, which we may blithely assume will happen when contraception ceases. Ironically, at this point the realisation emerges that the contraceptive precautions were unnecessary. Callan and Hennessy (1989) draw our attention to the perception of a lack of control over their lives which compounds the grief of infertile people.

The second factor unique to the grief of an infertile couple is the 'psychological roller-coaster' (Frank, 1984). Usually a person who is grieving experiences distress which gradually, either healthily or otherwise, is resolved and allows the person to continue their life. Because infertility and its investigations and treatment relate closely to the woman's cycle, the grief is regularly exacerbated when her menstrual period reminds her yet again that she has not conceived.

Aggravating factors

There are many factors which may 'rub salt into the wound' of a couple's infertility. The everyday assumptions which I have mentioned already are examples. Similarly, the well-meant but potentially cruel reminders from would-be grannies and aunties, which reflect this society's pronatalist attitudes and are referred to by Menning (1982) as 'needling'.

Infertility investigations may or may not provide a diagnostic label or indicate the cause of the problem, which in turn may suggest a solution. The absence of a diagnosis is the least satisfactory outcome (Frank, 1984). Having suggested that a solution may exist, I should look more closely at the possibility of such a solution. All too often solutions are no such thing, as many methods of 'assisted reproduction' carry implications which make them unacceptable to one or both of the couple (Mander & Whyte, 1985; Friedman, 1989), such as the involvement of a third party in articial insemination by donor (AID), or the lack of babies of a suitable ethnic background for adoption, or the underemphasised failure rates of the new reproductive technologies.

Effect on relationship

In the same way as men and women grieve any form of loss differently, the response of each partner to their infertility is likely to differ and generate tensions within the relationship. Brand (1989) shows that the differences which have been identified in grieving perinatal death (see

Chapter 6) apply equally in the couple's acceptance of their infertility. Although Brand does not go so far, it is likely that the resulting conflicts are also similar.

Because in the majority of couples the cause of infertility is attributable to just one of the partners, the other partner may inhibit their own grieving in order to be strong for their infertile mate (Frank, 1984), raising the likelihood of accusations of being callous or unfeeling and the potential for a deteriorating spiral in the relationship.

Summary

In this chapter I have looked at a range of childbearing situations which include an element of grieving. I have not been able to consider the minor griefs associated with a wrong-sex baby or a wrong birth, which did not happen as hoped. Although there are many common features in these grieving situations, there are also factors which are unique to each and which have implications for our care.

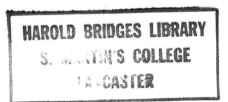

Chapter 4
Caring for the Grieving Mother

In Chapter 3 I considered the features of perinatal loss which may adversely affect the mother's grieving. Some of these features apply across the range of different forms of loss, whereas others are unique to specific situations. In this chapter I look at the implications of this knowledge for our care of the grieving mother. We should bear in mind that we may be caring for her at any stage in her loss. It may be as early as when her realisation of infertility first dawns or it may be during a subsequent pregnancy and birth.

An approach to care

I am looking, first, at general issues which influence our care, before focusing on the principles which determine our interventions when caring for the grieving mother. I focus on issues and principles, as I mentioned in the introduction, in order to avoid checklists or a cookbook format. Some, such as Brown (1992), suggest that checklists are appropriate in the care of the grieving mother; she recommends that her example is used alongside specific protocols in policy manuals. She maintains that this provides 'direction' for the management of births involving loss, although whether 'direction' is obligatory or advisory remains unclear.

Instruction may be appropriate, as envisaged by Oglethorpe (1989), when relatively junior staff are 'left to deal with perinatal casualties' and they lack either personal or occupational experience. Alternatively, a checklist may be a useful method of informing other members of staff of what has been achieved with the grieving mother, to avoid her having to repeat the same information at each change of shift.

The danger is that checklists may start out as guidance, but may become prescriptive 'tablets of stone', the original intention of which is long-forgotten (Lewis & Bourne, 1989). Similarly, checklists may result in a production-line approach, serving as a barrier to open caring and protecting us from painful psychological issues (Oglethorpe, 1989; Menzies, 1969; Mallinson, 1989).

Cautioning us to be wary of 'how-to' approaches to this mother's care, Leon (1992) recognises the place of general guidelines, but fears that they may inhibit 'emotionally engaging [with] parents'. As with many aspects of care, a routine approach, which a checklist generates, denies the uniqueness of both the mother's grief and the care which we are able to offer her. Avoiding a prescriptive approach is one reason for focusing on the principles influencing this mother's care. Additionally, the principles of care are relatively unchanging, while our provision of care may be affected by any number of factors, such as the individuals involved, the meaning they attach to the loss, and local circumstances.

The aims of care

When deciding how to offer care to the mother, it is necessary to ask first what we are trying to achieve. It is essential to take a long-term view of her care, so I endorse the aim of initiating mourning and minimising any impediments to grieving to help her recover healthily from her loss (Kirk, 1984; Bourne & Lewis, 1991).

General principles underpinning care

There are certain general principles which are applicable to many aspects of care but which assume particular significance in this context. I consider these before moving on to think about those principles which are unique to our care of the grieving mother.

Honesty and directness

The staff who are responsible for giving information about potential or actual loss may be tempted to skirt the issue in the hope of breaking bad news 'gently'. This sadly misguided intention results in compounding the mother's confusion rather than clarifying matters (Kirk, 1984). The mother seeking to have her worst fears either confirmed or refuted deserves this information with the minimum of delay. Although it has been argued that 'a little delay' may be acceptable (Lewis & Bourne, 1989), I cannot imagine that this benefits the mother. Whether the mother is made to wait 'to be told' pending the arrival of her partner, should not be an issue if she is well-supported during and after the giving of the bad news.

Who cares?

Whether the grieving mother should be cared for by staff specialising in bereavement relates to the argument discussed in Chapter 5 on who counsels. A Perinatal Crisis Support Group (Brown, 1992) was developed, as staff were experiencing 'difficulty'. The benefits of such specialised care to the mother are unevaluated. While surmising the advantages of care by highly-knowledgeable bereavement specialists, it is uncertain whether these outweigh continuity.

Cultural implications

Because our attitudes to death are inextricably bound up with our culture, it is essential to ensure that our help is culturally appropriate; in this context culture includes psychological, social and religious perspectives (Firth, 1993). Caring for a grieving mother who belongs to an ethnic minority is fraught with difficulties for staff who do not share her background.

Degree of 'westernisation'

Although we may assume that a certain appearance carries with it particular characteristics, our attention is drawn to the huge variation in 'westernisation' among a sample of Asian mothers in east London (Woollett & Dosanjh-Matwala, 1990). Assumptions often prove unfounded. In the same way as 'westernisation' varies, adherence to religious and traditional cultural values varies between individuals, requiring us to learn the preferences of those we care for.

Language

In their sample Woollett and Dosanjh-Matwala (1990) found that equal proportions (41%) spoke either 'extremely fluent' or 'little or no' English. Although our difficulty with others' languages is often a problem, in a grieving situation when verbal communication is fundamental, it becomes crucial.

The limited availability of translation aids and interpreters, may reflect racist attitudes endemic in UK society (Phoenix, 1990). Writing about the health experiences of black women Douglas (1992) emphasises the ethnocentric nature of the UK health care system, maintaining that the absence of relevant research perpetuates the problem. This lack of research on ethnic groups' health care definitely applies to perinatal loss.

Cultural assumptions

It may be difficult for us to recognise that some of the assumptions which we make about certain aspects of our lives, such as the relationships between men and women, may be little more than assumptions. It may be hard to accept others' views and attitudes if they differ. This may be a particular problem for those of us who live in parts of the country where we infrequently meet people from ethnic minorities.

This became apparent to me when I was caring for a mother whose two-day-old daughter died unexpectedly. The mother explained to me that ordinarily she would have found comfort by reading her Koran, but this was forbidden due to her being 'unclean'. For the same reason she was unable to attend her daughter's funeral, which generated non-comprehension and antipathy among some staff. Our limited under-standing of other ethnic groups emerged in my recent research (Mander, 1992d), when midwives gave me their impressions of some mothers' attitudes to loss:

Marie   They have completely different attitudes and things. Nobody under-stood [a bereaved mother's] need to grieve for this baby because with their religion it is completely different. They completely forget it and say 'Allah has taken it away and I'll be here to have another one'.

Ritual

Distinguishing religious observance from cultural ritual is neither easy nor necessary. Each of the major religions has significant rituals relating to caring for the deceased and for the grieving family, which carry meaning and provide much-needed help and support. Firth (1993) describes the washing and clothing of the body, the timing and form of the funeral and the prescribed mourning and social support. Jolly (1987) considers perinatal loss from the viewpoints of members of the Muslim, Hindu, Sikh, Christian and Jewish faiths. There are two aspects of care which merit particular attention. These are the acceptability of, first, a post mortem and, second, caring staff of another or no religion helping the mother.

Communication

The importance of communication in facilitating the processes of grieving is closely examined later, but the significance of this aspect of our care of the grieving mother cannot be overstated. Despite causing difficulty for some of us (Forrest, 1989), the carer's ability to listen may be more important than her ability to talk. However, the mother needs to be given information about a range of topics about grieving and more mundane things. How this information is given will determine whether it is accepted and implemented, so the information-giver must be con-stantly looking out for verbal and non-verbal cues which indicate acceptance or otherwise. It may be helpful at the beginning of a dis-cussion to review topics covered previously.

Worden (1992) warns us to avoid assumptions relating to the meaning of the pregnancy and its loss. While we may correctly assume that her loss constitutes an incapacitating tragedy, there may have been an element of ambivalence at some point in the pregnancy which, after the loss, engenders guilt and which may be magnified disproportionately by well-meant comments.

Communication with other staff for *their* benefit is discussed in Chapter 9, but I focus here on communication between staff for the mother's benefit. As I have mentioned already, staff taking over the mother's care at a shift change need information about topics which have been discussed with her. Better continuity may be achieved through practising primary midwifery or nursing, to reduce the number of new relationships which the mother is obliged to build (Kirk, 1984). But, regardless of how it is achieved, continuity and consistency of care are crucial.

Communication between staff is additionally important to protect the mother from the 'painful situations' (Forrest, 1989) arising when staff are ignorant of her loss. I can vouch that the pain is mutual, as I found when I answered a bell in a hectic labour ward to find a newly-arrived mother in the throes of giving birth. I helped appropriately, but was perplexed when she burst into tears on finding that she had a boy. The father explained that she had given birth to a stillborn boy two years earlier. Her painful memories were being resurrected while I felt anger and guilt at being unprepared.

Kennell *et al.* (1970) warn us of the dire consequences of lapses of interstaff communication, giving examples of bereaved mothers being told to feed their babies. In my recent study the relinquishing mothers frequently informed me of such lapses and the resulting sorrow. My label 'cockups' is appropriate. Alina, a poorly-supported 30-year-old, experienced a 'cockup' shortly after learning that she was pregnant:

Alina The student midwife read my notes which said I was devastated. She asked me how I was feeling and held my hand. She couldn't find the fetal heart using the monitor, so she got the sister. The sister bounced in saying 'What a lovely surprise and wasn't I pleased?' The student silently pointed to something in the notes and the sister looked aghast. She found the heartbeat and left – fast.

Davis *et al.* (1988) suggest that the mother's 'chart or door should be flagged' to identify her special situation. This suggestion is a sorry reflection on our individualisation of care.

Midwives' need for feedback emerged in my recent study:

Ottily You don't get any feedback about how they do afterwards.
Polly We did get a postcard from a bereaved mother who was extremely withdrawn and upset when she lost her baby. But she came to terms with it in a matter of a few months.
Annie Mums came back [to a midwives' study day] to talk about it and this provided us with feedback which we don't often get. We usually just get

their appreciation at the time and then maybe a letter of thanks a wee while later.

It is clearly necessary for us to learn more about how mothers perceive the value of the care we offer. Kirk (1984) suggests that the return visit to discuss the loss may be an opportunity for staff to glean feedback about the effects of their care, although improved continuity of care may be a better solution.

Tasks to facilitate grieving

There are certain tasks which, it has been suggested in the research and other literature, facilitate the mother's grieving. Our role as carers is to assist her in making progress with these tasks.

Recognising that she has had a baby

The research by Davidson (1977, see Chapter 3) suggests that the mother's confusion about who or what she has lost impedes her grieving.

Establishing the reality of her baby
The lack of reality of a baby who is 'unknown' in the usual sense is best resolved by the parents having contact with the baby (Kellner & Lake, 1986). This contact has been found to cause no adverse reactions and Davidson (1977) found that there is less psychiatric pathology among mothers who did see their babies.

Similarly, Alice Lovell (1983), during a research project involving 22 mothers who had lost a baby through perinatal death, found that of the 12 who saw their babies, none regretted having done so. These mothers were powerfully aware of their emotion-laden experience, but they thought that it was rewarding and appropriate. The 10 mothers who chose not to see their babies described their feelings as being 'in limbo' and their recollections featured regret.

Hermione Lovell *et al.* (1986) undertook a small retrospective study of bereaved mothers' views about their care around the time of a perinatal death. Twenty mothers were interviewed for up to 90 minutes about three years after their loss. The mothers were still finding difficulty understanding their loss, although those for whom it was their second perinatal loss fared better; their previous experience had taught them the difficulty of grieving for an unknown baby and they resolved to ensure that, at least, their grieving progressed as they wished. These previously-bereaved mothers were able to be assertive in making contact with the baby and in arranging the funeral.

Women should be able to have an optimal experience of loss without having to lose a second baby in order to do so. For such an experience the mother requires information which will allow her to make an informed decision about, for example, making contact with her baby. The information and encouragement about contact which midwives in my recent study were prepared to give to mothers was variable:

Bessie I'd never force anyone though. I certainly would not want to cuddle anything that was dead myself. If that is how she feels she can look at it in the cot and that is fine, or she can look at it the next day and that is fine.

Gay I think they should see the wee one . . . but they might not think they want to hold it. I think the midwife should really try and encourage them 'cos they'll regret it later on. Y'know they'll feel it's not really happened to them. But I don't mean that you actually force them to look at it. You know you should just sort of advise them and then it's up to them.

Hattie I don't think it's our duty to keep on bringing it up ... I don't think we should be bullying them into doing what we think's best.

Amy Its very much a personal thing . . . You'd always give her the chance – ask her if she wants to see the baby and let her cuddle it after it's born. Or if she doesn't want to you could take the baby away from her, give it a wash and then ask her again, and then about half an hour or an hour afterwards ask whether she wants to see the baby.

Although the midwives were generally happy to offer some encouragement for the mother to make contact with her baby, they were reluctant to 'strongly encourage' contact (Kirk, 1984).

Although the value of contact is well-established by research, we are not told how much encouragement or pressure the mothers were under to make contact or whether this affected their perception of the contact.

In his commentary on two case-studies of mothers who had declined contact, Leon (1992), rather than endorsing the orthodoxy of contact, advocates the empowerment of the mother to do what is right for her. He maintains that the helplessness engendered by being forced into certain behaviours may be as painful as any feelings of loss. Leon's misgivings about enforced contact are echoed by Lewis and Bourne (1989) on the grounds that procedures may become unthinkingly institutionalised and devoid of meaning. Like Mallinson (1989) and Bessie and Amy (above), these writers plead for the mother to have time to consider and opportunities to reconsider her decision.

The place of the cot

During my recent research I came to appreciate midwives' need to help the grieving mother accept the reality of her baby and her loss. Although the midwives were keen to encourage contact with the baby and were happy to be open in their communication with the grieving mother, they regarded the presence of the cot with concern, if not distaste. Unlike other equipment which has multiple uses, the cot has only one use and that is for holding a baby. This issue was first raised by Irene in response to a question about the birthing room:

Irene   The cot is always removed from the room before this woman goes in. It would dominate the room if it was present. Even with a couple with a normal healthy baby there is always a comment about the cot when they first go into the room. I would not like keeping the cot in the delivery room. It would probably be too distressing to the parents, although I am speculating about that. There was one woman, though, who refused to hold her baby, so I had to put the baby down onto the trolley while I delivered the third stage. It was really odd having to put the baby on the trolley, I didn't like having to do it. I had to wheel the baby out with all the rubbish. It was so clinical and cold having to put the baby on to the trolley that time.

Clearly the presence of the cot is viewed sufficiently negatively by some midwives to cause them to tolerate much inconvenience to avoid it. But Josie took a more flexible approach:

Josie   The cot sometimes stays in, sometimes it is out. I sometimes leave it in and if the woman objects then I'll take it out, but you need to put the baby somewhere. It depends on the individual mother, whether they want the cot left in or not, or whether they then hope you leave the cot there.

Thus, as well as its practical use, the presence of the cot assumes a symbolic significance, which may encourage denial.

Kerrie   I think it's best just to take the cot out. I think it's the right thing to do, possibly because I feel embarrassed in that situation myself. I wouldn't like a cot to be there.

Kerrie's discomfort leads us to ask whether the cot usually being occupied by a living baby serves to remind us of our failure in helping this woman achieve successful childbirth. Alternatively, does the removal of the cot constitute a denial of the baby's existence and reduce the birth to a mere surgical procedure?

Recognising that her baby has been born

I vividly recall the care of the grieving mother in labour in the 1960s involving the administration of large amounts of 'sedative', actually narcotic analgesic, drugs (Klaus & Kennell, 1982a). This regime, feasible because there was no risk of neonatal respiratory depression, was intended to block the mother's memories of the event, probably, for the staff's benefit (Kohner, 1985; Mallinson, 1989). Remembering this, I become concerned when 'generous' pain relief is recommended (Adams & Prince, 1990). Although I have argued the right of each mother to effective pain control and to feel the amount of pain which she wants to feel (Mander, 1992a), all involved should be clear about the rationale and use the appropriate route and medication.

If recollections of her experience are blocked for the heavily-sedated mother, the mother who gives birth under general anaesthesia has even fewer memories and greater confusion (Lewis, 1976). I would question whether the mother is similarly denied memories and opportunities to help her work through her grief by the prescription of tranquillisers postnatally (Lovell *et al.*, 1986).

Realising that she is a mother

The limited physical and visual contact between the mother and baby may cause her and others to either forget or deny that she is a mother. Lovell (1984) suggests that birth and death, being perceived as positive and negative events respectively, may be seen as cancelling each other out and generating a 'non-event'. The result is that she is 'stripped' of her motherhood, which aggravates her feelings of the non-reality of the event. We are able, through our care, to remind her that although she may not have a baby with her, she has still become a mother. Thus, 'routine' postnatal care (see below) will in this mother assume extra significance, such as the community visits reaffirming her motherhood (Mallinson, 1989).

A crucial component of motherhood lies in caring for the baby. By giving the mother opportunities to behave as ordinary mothers do, such as by cuddling her baby and by bathing and dressing the baby, it will be reinforced that she was able to show her love by mothering her baby, albeit only briefly (Awoonor-Renner, 1993). A physiological process such as lactation (see below) may also serve to reinforce her motherhood if she does not have her baby with her, or she may be able to provide breast milk if her baby is dangerously ill in the neonatal unit.

Recognising that her baby is dead

The interventions discussed above to confirm that the baby has been born apply equally to helping the mother to recognise that her baby is dead. Her recognition will be facilitated by providing full and factual information about her baby's death. Because she may be unable to take in all the information when it is first provided verbally, it should also be given in writing to allow her to return to it and review what she was told. The reality of the death will be recognised by the use of the rituals which ordinarily happen when death occurs in her culture; such as caring for the body, mourning, funeral rites and providing social support.

Memories

The significance of memories is made clear by Allingham (1952):

'Mourning is not forgetting, it is an undoing. Every minute tie has to be untied and something permanent and valuable recovered and assimilated from the knot'.

Much of our grieving depends on having memories (Mallinson, 1989) on which we can focus our thoughts, either alone or with others, in order to adjust our view of the person who is lost. We come to terms with our good and not-so-good recollections of them, while accepting that we have no more opportunities to interact with them directly. In this way we can grieve and eventually become reconciled to our loss. In the absence of tangible memories, any focus for our grief is lacking, which may inhibit its progress.

Creating memories

The interventions which we use to help the mother create memories on which to focus her grief are explained by Lewis (1976). They comprise largely the rituals ordinarily associated with death, such as laying out the body, viewing the body and holding a funeral; the burial or cremation serves to both help create memories and give a physical focus to help long-term grieving.

Lewis and Page (1978) describe the interventions they used to create memories of her stillborn son for a mother with pathological grief due to failure to mourn. They reconstructed the non-event by 'bringing the baby back to death' to enable the mother to remember, relive and belatedly grieve her loss. As carers in the maternity area we aim to promote healthy grieving by creating memories as the birth and subsequent events unfold, rather than having to intervene retrospectively to resolve pathological grief.

Tangible, durable mementoes serve as a focus for grief as well as confirming the reality of the event. One example, photos, should not fade (Mallinson, 1989); an old grainy photo may be a sufficient reminder as time passes.

The baby as an individual

Recognising the baby as a unique individual helps the mother to differentiate her dead baby from any others and from her own fantasies and narcissistic dreams. We help her to establish the individuality of her baby by focusing on any unique characteristics as well as differences from any siblings. Even though it is not legally required, we encourage the mother to name her lost child, as this provides a focus, as well as helping communication with others (Klaus & Kennell, 1982a; SANDS, 1991). In a situation in which the mother may feel that she has little to contribute, being able to give her baby a name becomes significant, as I learned from the relinquishing mothers in my recent study:

Iona   But Andrea had always been my favourite name and I wanted to give her something and that was all I could give her. So I gave her the name Andrea.

In a study of perinatal loss associated with the founding of SANDS, Lewis (1978) found that over 60% of her sample of 80 parents considered that having their baby recognised as a real person was their major concern; naming the baby and using this may facilitate recognition.

Making the birth as good an experience as possible

Although making a perinatal loss into a happy event is out of the question, it can become at least an experience which the mother is able to recall with satisfaction through having completed it with dignity (Kohner, 1985). To do this the grieving mother should be encouraged to participate actively in the birth, as should any mother (Mallinson, 1989).

Although, in the past, medication has been used to sedate the grieving mother for the convenience of the staff (see above), Dyer (1992) recommends that the mother should, if she wants to, be able to feel the pain of labour. This may correspond with her 'emotional pain' and perhaps also give her as complete an experience of labour as possible. Sensation of her pain may allow her some sense of satisfaction or achievement so that she is able to look back and think 'At least I managed that'.

Fathoming the complexity of this event

The psychological work which the grieving mother faces is awesome; she must disentangle and grieve for a confusing mix of potential and actual phenomena. She has to separate out the threads of dreams and reality, of herself and her baby, of this loss and previous and future losses. Completing this mammoth task is helped by sharing the load, and being listened to has been identified as the most fundamental need at this time (Standish, 1982). While listening to her we encourage the mother to articulate her dreams about her baby and help her to think about the meaning of her baby and her loss.

Lovell *et al.* (1986) highlighted the mother's difficulty in finding suitable people with whom she could unburden herself; senior staff lacked the time to spend listening, while younger staff were considered too inexperienced and lacked the personal touch.

The importance of listening is emphasised by Davis *et al.* (1988) as a way of reducing the mother's isolation. Listening and a reduction of isolation were identified by Yates (1972) as the overwhelming needs of grieving mothers. However, the difficulty of listening to her speaking angrily or guiltily should not be underestimated, especially if her anger is partly directed at carers, as we may find it hard not to react to what we may perceive as personal attacks.

The difficulty of making time to listen emerged in my recent study. The midwives told me of the strategies they used to ensure that they were not disturbed while with a grieving mother. They were aware that, although they might make time to be with the mother for an hour, say between 14.00 and 15.00, that might not be the time when the mother felt like 'opening-up'.

The mother needs to be able to talk about what it is that she feels she has lost without the listener trying to change the subject or backing off. Hermione Lovell *et al.* (1986) found that previously-bereaved mothers (see above) were able to satisfy their need to talk through their loss.

Alice Lovell (1983) draws our attention to a discrepancy which confronts a grieving mother. Ordinarily each of us has some need to communicate with our fellow beings, if only about the weather, but at times of crisis, our need to share our feelings is increased. The grieving mother, however, is faced with the prospect of not even being allowed to satisfy her usual need to talk, let alone her increased 'quota'. This constitutes an 'ironic' discrepancy which aggravates her feelings of isolation and rejection.

Although we are unable to know what her loss means to her, we assume that it is significant. This helps us to give her opportunities to work out what the meaning is to her.

I needed to remember this when I was caring in the postnatal ward for a new mother whose growth-retarded son had been born at 26 weeks. She seemed calm, but told me repeatedly that no-one was feeding her dog. She was reluctant to see her son. I explained how ill he was and that it was all right for her to be sad. She began to cry and talk of her hopes for him. A little while later the NNU staff asked for her to go to see him and she was able to hold him while he died.

As well as listening, we need to give her information, including telling her that we are available to be there and listen.

Preparing to face the future

Although the grieving mother may have difficulty envisaging a future in the absence of what was a major part of her, we may encourage her to relate her experience of loss to her future life.

Grieving

By telling her about grieving we are able to help her to understand the process by which she will eventually become reconciled to her loss. Information (Cook & Oltjenbruns, 1989) will help her to know that grief is appropriate, that it is painful, enduring and unique and that her grief may include negative feelings which may shock her. Davis *et al.* (1988)

suggest that by emphasising that such frightening responses have been felt by other grieving mothers, we are able to reduce her sense of isolation.

She should be told, as far as possible, what will and what will not help her grief and be forewarned that the hurtful 'have another' comments are not meant unkindly and are best forgotten. It may help her to know that her experience of loss may change her and those close to her in ways which are unpredictable and possibly unwelcome, but such changes are not unique to grief.

Pitfalls
As well as preparing her to cope with the healthy development of her grief, warnings about certain times and events may prevent her from feeling that she is taking 'two steps back' when they confront her.

The post mortem
The request for a post mortem may shock a mother who considers that her baby has been through enough already (Laurent, 1993; Mallinson, 1989).

The funeral
A young mother with no experience of bereavement may regard the funeral as a macabre irrelevance, but an explanation of the short- and long-term benefits may help her to decide whether and how it should be organised (Mallinson, 1989).

The nursery
Well-meaning but unthinking family may have already 'dealt with' the nursery, but if not she may appreciate the opportunity, when she feels ready, to complete this 'unfinished business'.

Anniversaries
At anniversaries she may be disappointed at her reaction. But when she recollects the joy of, for example, her first scan, her reaction may seem less disproportionate. Others' difficulties are aggravated by some of the anniversaries, such as the conception, being 'hidden' (i.e. only the mother/couple know about it) (Mallinson, 1989).

Future childbearing
Future childbearing (see Chapter 12) should be mentioned to the mother as she may feel a need for a 'replacement child'.

Finding support
The benefits of support to those who are grieving have been established

in the context of perinatal death (Forrest *et al.*, 1982) as has the difficulty of resolving grieving in the absence of social support (Helmrath & Steinitz, 1978). I look at some issues relating to lay support in Chapter 11.

Being available

The supportive nature of the carer's company emerges in the work of Lovell (1983) and I have already observed (see above) the need for us to be available for the mother. Our presence may involve listening, information-giving, sharing her tears or just being present. Finding the right balance between being companionable and being intrusive worried the midwives in my recent study:

> *Kay* I think that it's a very important thing to give them some privacy. If you're outside with the door open or within shouting distance, they don't need you to be there all the time . . . a careful decision to make. Also you don't want them to feel that they've just been abandoned – gone away – nobody cares. You've got to tell them 'I'm over the other side'.

The role of the midwife in providing social support for a grieving mother has been established recently in a study of 509 mothers, half of whom had experienced previous pregnancy loss (Rajan & Oakley, 1993). The research midwives gave non-directive social support tailored to the individual mother. This low-tech intervention helped the mothers' emotional health on both a short-term and a long-term basis. The mothers were able to deal with unresolved grief and to prepare themselves to cope with an anxiety-provoking pregnancy. Many of the mothers became more self-confident and reasserted control over their lives.

Family support

Because the family is likely to be providing support on a longer-term basis, they need to be involved in the mother's short-term care and her teaching about matters such as grief, self-care, the development of grief (see Chapter 6; Klaus & Kennell, 1982a). They also need to understand their own grief as well as hers (Davis *et al.*, 1988), partly to help them to avoid well-meant but hurtful comments.

Open and honest communication between family members enables them to share their reactions to their loss; this may happen despite a previously 'closed' system of communication (Benfield *et al.*, 1978).

Other support

Family and community support may be forthcoming in the religious or cultural rituals associated with death, such as the funeral (Kirk, 1984).

The grieving mothers interviewed by Lovell (1983) found that the 'community' is less caring and comforting than its name implies, leading to Lovell's conclusion that the mother might be better supported if she remains in the maternity unit longer. These mothers would also have welcomed the support of a self-help group, but only half of the sample were aware of their existence. On the basis of these data she suggests that the health visitor has an important role to play in the long-term care of the grieving mother.

Being in control

Her untimely loss may convince the mother that her control over her life has diminished.

Learned helplessness is a person's response to their own inability to control their circumstances, although whether it occurs will depend on their interpretation of their loss. This term is used to describe the debilitated behaviour of a person who is subjected to some form of assault (such as electric shocks applied in a laboratory) over which they have no control. Learned helplessness comprises three main components, which are deficits in functioning:

(1) the deficit in motivation comprises the person's inability to initiate any voluntary responses – on the assumption that to do so would be futile.
(2) the cognitive deficit causes the person to have difficulty learning in future that responses may produce outcomes. Theirs is the difficulty of unlearning something that they have learned by painful experience.
(3) the depressed affect results from the conviction that you cannot change anything.

These features are based on the expectation that what has happened in the past will continue to apply in the future, that is the absence of control is unalterable (Garber & Seligman, 1980).

Perinatal loss gives rise to feelings of personal helplessness and pathological grief if the mother believes that there is something she could have done which might have prevented the loss of her baby, such as resting more or eating better (Stroebe & Stroebe, 1987). Our role in enabling this mother to retain both a sense of and actual control relates largely to the information which she is given. Accurate information and possibly a post mortem report should show her that feelings of self-blame are inappropriate. Additionally she needs information about the choices which are open to her and information on which she can base her decisions.

Choices and control

For some mothers *induction of labour* may be recommended, and she decides whether and when this happens (see Chapter 3).

There may be a choice about the *place of birth*, although it may be only the location within the maternity unit (Kohner, 1985); depending on her condition, she may have other alternatives.

I have already considered the mother's decision about *contact* with her baby (see above).

The *mother's accommodation* after a birth in a maternity unit has been the focus of much attention, although the midwives in my recent study were unaware of the mother's choice:

Amy   The decision is made by nursing staff and hospital policy. Here they always come to antenatal 'cos antenatal is the only place with single rooms. But when I worked up at . . . they went to postnatal because postnatal had single rooms there and they were a postnatal lady.
Hilary   She has a single room so that she'll be protected from the other mothers.

Hughes (1986) indicates that other mothers were not averse to being alongside a bereaved mother, suggesting that midwives' anxiety about other mothers' actively harmful role is unjustified. These findings are reinforced by the comments of relinquishing mothers who found help among other mothers:

Lena   Actually the women [in the big ward] were OK. And they used to mother me. They realised I was just a kid. They were OK to me. I think before I had the baby I wanted to be in a room on my own. I didn't want anyone to see me. But I was glad really that I was 'cos even though it was [a big ward] the women were all nice. We were all just girls together. They done their exercises and had a bit of a giggle and they all were nice to me. They all sorta looked after me.

These data lead to the conclusion that the grieving mother as well as other mothers would be happy to share accommodation, but the staff who make or at least implement these decisions have other concerns, such as midwives' anxiety that the grieving mother would be disturbed by babies' crying. The midwives were unable to contemplate the possibility that the avoidance of other mothers and babies might be associated with a denial of the loss.

The midwives were reluctant to burden the mother with mundane decisions about her care. These decisions include the type of ward in which she is cared for, the size of room which she should occupy or, if larger, the mothers with whom she should share it (pregnant women, new mothers or mothers of babies in NNU). Such decisions were attributed to unit policy. Sharing a room with another mother was considered to be unhelpful for the grieving mother, as the onset of her mourning is delayed and her support system may be impaired.

Midwives' reluctance to allow or encourage the grieving mother to make decisions about her accommodation is unfortunate, as the choices open to her and her control over her situation are being limited.

Lovell (1984) identified feelings of isolation and rejection among her sample of grieving mothers, which related to being cared for in single rooms. The relinquishing mothers I interviewed referred to themselves as like a 'ghost at the banquet'. Lovell found that hospital staff encountered difficulty in caring for the grieving mother appropriately and as a result *transfer her home* 'with undue haste'. Although the midwives in my study maintained that the grieving mother was in control of how long she stayed in hospital, their examples did not bear this out:

Hilary   I think that as long as everything is all right she should be able to go home the next day. She should have as short a stay in hospital as possible.

Izzy   In this hospital their stay is short. It's very much up to the patient as to when she wants to go home. They're really pretty flexible about it. Some people would like to go home quickly. If they deliver in the morning then some of them will go home that evening. If they deliver during the night, they maybe go home the following afternoon.

Lucy   But we usually tend to let them go home as soon as they want to go home, we would allow them to go home as long as they are physically fit. And that seems to work best as long as we can see that they are coping with the grief as well.

Although lip service is being paid to the mother assuming control, the reality needs investigation. Gohlish's exploratory study (1985) involved interviews with 15 mothers of stillborn babies to identify the nursing behaviours which were most helpful. Her 20 behavioural statements focused on the mother assuming control over her situation. But those statements which the mothers thought 'most helpful' clearly related to control:

(1) Recognise when I want to talk about my baby.
(2) Allow me to stay as long or as short a time in hospital as I wish.
(3) Let me decide if I want a single room or main ward.
(4) Ask me if I want a photograph of my baby.
(5) Explain to me that I may produce milk.
(6) Explain to me that I can see the baby after several days.
(7) Give me pain relief as often as needed.

Grieving mothers felt the need to assume or be allowed more control over their care. Unfortunately my study, which was completed seven years later, fails to show that her findings are being utilised.

Obtaining the care that a new mother needs

As suggested already in the context of care in labour, midwifery care seeks to prevent those problems which would create harmful memories and which would prevent the mother focusing her grief on her loss. The need for information, which applies to all mothers, becomes more significant for the grieving mother who is trying to make sense of the confusing situation and conflicting emotions which beset her.

Home visits by the midwife
In view of the haste with which the mother is likely to go home, her care by the community midwife assumes greater significance. Home visits were found to be appreciated for both their physical and their psychological value (Lovell, 1983; Cooper, 1980).

These observations contrast with those by Hermione Lovell *et al.* (1986), whose respondents disliked home visits for two reasons. First, the personal characteristics of the midwives were unacceptable, in that they were 'very cut off, very professional'. The second factor which may not be unrelated is the difficulty which the grieving mother has in understanding why the midwife visits her, when she has no baby. This may be exacerbated by the midwife not being aware of the mother's loss. Uncertainty about the midwife's role had been faced by a community midwife I interviewed:

Ginnie   Sometimes they can be a bit antagonistic, y'know the first couple of visits and 'Do you have to come to see me? I don't need a midwife.' And you sit down with them and try and explain that you are there to make sure that she is alright and everything is returning to normal . . .

Lactation
One of the most helpful nursing behaviours (see above) in Gohlish's study (1985) was 'Explain to me that I may produce milk'. A mother may assume that if she has no baby with her, nothing will be produced with which to feed it. Our increasing knowledge of the physiology of lactation shows us that the mother's thought processes are crucially important; so that thinking about her baby has an effect similar to the baby suckling. It is, thus, hardly surprising that the grieving mother produces milk, as recounted by one of Lovell's respondents:

Fiona   Walking down the road and seeing a pram with a baby in it, I'd have to go home and change my tee-shirt, it'd be soaked. The milk kept coming for months after.

Fiona obviously regarded her lactation negatively, but we must question whether this need invariably be the case. Lewis and Bourne (1989) suggest that it may be comforting for the mother to know that, her baby would have been well-fed if alive.

Summary

Much of the literature reminds us of the bad old days when the 'rugger pass' technique of surreptitiously hustling the baby out of the mother's presence prevailed. In thinking about our care of this mother we must be wary of forcing a new, perhaps more liberal, orthodoxy on her (Lewis & Bourne, 1989). I have argued in this chapter that our role is to facilitate the mother's healthy grieving, which is assisted by her having a positive childbearing experience to recall. To achieve this the mother should be encouraged to assume some control of her experience; which, in turn, is dependent on her being provided with accurate research-based information about interventions and outcomes. Unfortunately such information is incomplete.

Chapter 5
Bereavement Counselling

I occasionally find myself wondering what bereavement counselling is about. Having begun with a very precise focus, it may have snowballed to become a panacea. My anxiety relates to the fervour with which it is recommended, the variability of the recipients, the wide-ranging activities included and the variety of practitioners; leading to the conclusion that it is 'all things to all people'. In this chapter I consider the nature of bereavement counselling, who is involved and its relevance following perinatal loss. As in counselling literature, I use the term 'client'.

What bereavement counselling does and does not involve

Bereavement counselling and grief therapy are not easily distinguishable (Cook & Dworkin, 1992), perhaps due to sloppy terminology or, alternatively, to common areas, such as the client having been bereaved. The large area of overlap between bereavement counselling and therapy increases the risk of confusion. The difference is found in the client (Worden, 1992); in bereavement counselling the client is being supported through uncomplicated grieving, whereas grief therapy treats pathological grief.

Counselling is defined in terms of source of control in a nursing context, when the counsellor acts merely as a facilitator to help the client identify and 'sort out his or her own problems' (Burnard & Morrison, 1991). Likewise, Barker (1983) emphasises the relative inactivity of the counsellor when, following a multicentre study of counselling for bereaved elderly, he defines it as 'friendly listening'. Epstein (1989) uses similar functional terms when he focuses on the emotional and practical support which counselling provides to reduce the pain of bereavement.

The facilitative role mentioned already may not always be regarded as relevant (Raphael-Leff, 1991). Bereavement counselling to *prevent* psychiatric and psychosomatic disorders has been researched (Parkes, 1980; Forrest *et al*., 1982). Although counselling does not aim to *treat* pathological grief, it may constitute a preventative rather than a therapeutic approach to disordered grieving. Unlike the supportive approaches mentioned previously, tertiary treatment or grief therapy comprises active and significant interventions to bring about emotional and cognitive changes in the client (Cook & Dworkin, 1992)

Evaluation

As with any form of care, when we recommend bereavement counselling we should be certain that the client is given full information about what it is as well as any side-effects. This information is only available if the intervention has been fully researched.

In Parkes' (1980) review of authoritative research (Raphael, 1977; Gerber *et al.*, 1975; Polak *et al.*, 1975), he concludes that bereavement counselling services reduce the risk of disordered grieving. The classical experimental design was utilised in these studies; people identified as bereaved through official sources were recruited and randomly allocated to either the counselling or the non-counselling group. After counselling was completed, health measures were applied to assess any differences. That counselling causes more problems than it solves (Freud cited in Worden, 1992) is not supported by this evidence.

Cameron and Parkes (1983) used a similar design to research the effects of bereavement counselling; they found similarly effective results, but were implicitly critical of the chosen design. These researchers regretted their inability to identify *which* components of the counselling programme were effective.

We may criticise the use of the classical experimental design in more general terms, to the extent that these studies do not establish whether the actual counselling made any difference, because the fact of *some* intervention may have been sufficient to produce the favourable results. At such a vulnerable time the bereaved person may be grateful for *any* form of human contact, whether or not it helps her adjustment to her loss.

Such alteration in the subject's behaviour because of her involvement in a study, or the Hawthorne effect (Carter, 1991), could have been avoided by amending the design. If, instead of having only two groups of subjects, the researchers had introduced a third 'other intervention' group, they would have been able to ascertain whether counselling was responsible for the improved outcomes. The ethical implications of any such 'other intervention' would need attention, but learning a neutral subject, such as a language, would satisfy the research requirements.

Unlike other studies evaluating bereavement counselling, Forrest *et al.* (1982) focused on perinatal loss. The sample, interviewed long-itudinally, comprised 25 mothers of stillborn babies and 25 whose babies had died as newborns. They found that counselled mothers recovered from their grief quicker than the contrast group. The difference was significant at 6 months, but not at 14 months.

The benefits of these research projects focus on the long-term health outcomes of bereaved people. Little attention is given to the client's experience of counselling, unlike a less authoritative study by Barker (1983) in which general satisfaction and occasional gratitude is reported.

The need to learn of the client's view derives from the attrition rate in Forrest's study, which may have been due to a variety of factors. Only 16 out of the 25 (64%) of the supported group and 19 (75%) of the unsupported group agreed to be interviewed at 6 months. By 14 months 20 (40%) of the original sample were unavailable for interview; unfortunately we are not told which group they were in. Although bereavement counselling is not intended to be enjoyable, this loss from the study may indicate dissatisfaction and needs investigation.

The client

Clearly, because resources are finite, whether counselling is available is determined by what it includes. If counselling comprises non-professional support to maintain healthy grieving, it may be available to many. On the other hand, if it is regarded as a preventive intervention, professionals skilled in psychotherapeutic techniques may be needed, with clear resource implications.

Worden (1992) suggests indications for counselling; either the person may actually have become 'stuck' in their grief or carers using 'at-risk' criteria may seek to prevent problems occurring. The route by which clients find their way into counselling has been identified by Barker (1983) as a combination of the two, involving a 'watching brief' being kept by certain professionals, such as GPs and HVs (health visitors), and referral of those identified as at risk.

The counselling process

While it is neither appropriate nor possible to detail the skills and techniques of counselling here, there are certain essential features which help us to understand it.

The counsellor's 'way of being'

There are three essential characteristics (Lendrum & Syme, 1992) which a counsellor should have which may differ from our usual responses to painful situations:

- **Acceptance** of the uniqueness of the client's hurt, and being non-judgemental of her feelings.
- **Empathy**, comprising the ability to enter the world of the client

without the barriers of pity or fear. Morse *et al.* (1992) probe the extent of empathy by focusing on the nurse's self- or client-centredness and whether her empathy is intuitive or learned.

- **Congruence** or the self-awareness in the counsellor which allows her to be genuine and accepting of herself. Through her behaviour, she conveys acceptance to her client, as mentioned already.

These characteristics are crucial to effective counselling as they provide an emotional environment in which healing and growth are nurtured. Although these characteristics may occur naturally in some of us, others may have to learn them during a counselling course. A supervisor helps a counsellor to maintain these characteristics, ensuring that counselling remains effective.

Tasks to work through grief

There are certain tasks with which the counsellor provides encouragement, in order to work through grief, in addition to creating an appropriate grieving environment (Worden, 1992:42).

- **Actualising the loss**   Through talking about the death and its circumstances and by focusing on tangible manifestations, such as the grave, the reality of the loss becomes evident.
- **Identifying and expressing feelings**   Because of the pain which they bring us, the client may resist identifying and expressing her feelings. The counsellor encourages articulation of anger, guilt, sorrow, anxiety and helplessness.
- **Living without the dead person**   This may be particularly difficult when roles are complementary and there may be gaps in many aspects of functioning. The counsellor may have to assist practically to show the client her own ability.
- **Relocating emotions**   Relocating the emotions invested in the dead person helps the client to realise that, although her relationship with the dead person was unique, her emotional energy may eventually be redirected into other, new relationships.
- **Allowing time**   By providing time to grieve the counsellor helps the client to recognise the gradual process by which we reconcile ourselves to loss. Memories persist in returning and causing emotional reactions for a surprisingly long time.
- **Recognising 'normal' grief behaviour**   The client should be reassured that her preoccupation, for example, does not indicate a nervous breakdown.
- **Continuing support**   The counsellor's continuing support is within the contract negotiated during the first meeting (Epstein, 1989),

although contacts tend to become less frequent before the counselling relationship is due to end.

- **Identifying defences and coping mechanisms** The counsellor should help the client to work out which defences and coping mechanisms are helpful, as opposed to those, such as drugs or alcohol, which may impair grieving (Worden, 1992:51). Other differently harmful defences include immersion in work and other forms of denial (Ridley, 1993). These defences protect us by diverting our attention away from painful events on a short term basis, but prevent effective grieving if they persist. These defences may only be breached if there is confidence in the counsellor.

Problems

Identifying pathology and making a referral is necessary when unforeseen problems are encountered. A grief therapist and psychotherapeutic interventions may prevent the situation from deteriorating.

The counsellor

Having briefly considered what happens during counselling, it is useful to think about the people who offer this form of help. By way of introducing his literature review, Parkes (1980) lists the three groups of counsellors whose functioning has been evaluated:

- professional services by trained personnel
- voluntary services using trained volunteers with professional support
- self-help or mutual support groups (see Chapter 11).

Although voluntary services contribute hugely to counselling services generally (Barker, 1983; Epstein, 1989), their input into perinatal bereavement counselling services is less. For this reason I focus on midwives and nurses as counsellors.

The suitability of midwives and nurses to be counsellors has been questioned (Burnard & Morrison, 1991) because essential attitudes (see above), summarised as 'client-centredness', may not easily fit into traditional nursing thought processes.

Burnard and Morrison surveyed the 'client-centredness' of a mixed sample of 142 qualified nurses. Their opportunistic sample was recruited through attendance at counselling skills workshops. These authors draw our attention to the potential unrepresentativeness of the sample, but fail to recognise that, because these nurses were enhancing their counselling skills, they were probably *more* client-centred in their approach than most nurses.

Using an instrument with a maximum score of 70, the nurses

assessed their own client-centredness. Their scores ranged from 22 to 67 with an overall mean score of 39, which the researchers interpret as a 'lack of a marked tendency towards client-centredness'.

They contrast this finding of 'prescriptive' attitudes with the frequent exhortations for patient autonomy. They then suggest that client-centredness, because of its time-consuming reflective approach, may be less than appropriate in a busy clinical setting. The authors do not link their findings to nurses' ability to be client-centred in their counselling, although it is tempting to assume that the attitudes reflected in the questionnaire apply more generally than in the clinical situations which the authors discussed.

Counselling following sudden death

Because of the limited research-based material on perinatal bereavement counselling, I draw on research which has some common aspects, such as untimeliness.

The establishment of a bereavement counselling service in an accident and emergency department (A&E) is recounted by Yates *et al.* (1993). The nurse-counsellor's educative function is emphasised, as is her ongoing support of relatives who are considered to be at risk of complicated grieving. Because the nurse-counsellor spends a finite time in A&E, a group of other senior nurses have been trained to offer a similar service. The nurse-counsellor provides emotional support for her colleagues as well as liaising with other professional groups.

This account suggests that, in contrast to the findings of Burnard and Morrison (1991), nursing support may be appropriate in bereavement. Ellison (1990) describes her experience of being a bereavement nurse-counsellor based in A&E and the marked extent to which she implements a 'client-centred' approach. She recounts how she facilitated the development of self-help counselling (Parkes, 1980) by making contact with 'The Compassionate Friends' and establishing a group.

A midwife interviewed in my recent study envisaged a similar scheme in the maternity area – also an emergency service:

Deidre   I think a counsellor would be quite important. I think it would be very good if somebody was trained and was able to counsel these women before they left the hospital and then could visit them in the community. She would need special training and counselling skills which would make it practical for her to be the one . . . it would be very hard for somebody to do that as a full-time job. It would be very emotionally demanding.

Woodward *et al.* (1985), using a social work perspective, recount the counselling service which they established for parents losing a child through sudden infant death syndrome (SIDS). As in Yates *et al.*

(above), the service originated in A&E. Woodward describes the importance of the initial assessment in helping parents sort out a range of mainly practical problems. Unlike Ellison though, Woodward recommends that appointments be made for home visits, because of the tendency of young bereaved families to be away from home. Longer-term counselling focused largely on family problems such as marital difficulties and helping surviving children. As observed already, the children who were worst affected were those whose parents were coping less well.

The midwife Deidre, like some writers, mentions the extra support which is likely to be needed by personnel who undertake bereavement counselling duties (Woodward *et al.*, 1985; Epstein, 1989; Barker, 1983). The lack of such support is regretted by a midwife following a tragic stillbirth; she regrets that only lip-service is paid to openness, asking 'Who counsels the counsellor?' (Anon, 1991).

Perinatal bereavement counselling

Ginnie I don't think just one person should do all [the counselling] though. A sister was employed in – Maternity Hospital and she was the counselling sister and it was too much for one person. It needs two to share because you are only human too, you're going to get distressed.

Like Ginnie in my recent study and the sadly anonymous midwife above, Druery (1992) identifies the need for emotional support in her role as a bereavement support midwife. Initially a psychologist provided support, but mutual support has become established by Druery and her two colleagues. Although avoiding the title 'counsellor' due to the lack of a qualification, her role in supporting parents by listening and seeking to prevent further problems is reminiscent of the counselling functions already mentioned. Druery demonstrates the educational component of her role in the teaching of students and information-giving to parents. She details how bereavement support is integrated into her midwifery role, but her difficulty in moving between the two roles produces a sense of 'schizophrenia'.

While Druery's appointment developed from a management in-itiative, Collins (1986) began her counselling role during a survey of perinatal deaths. Her induction as a research midwife included learning about interviewing and bereavement counselling and, like Ellison (1990), she has built links with self-help groups.

The relevance of counselling skills to midwives whose job description includes support is clear. For three reasons we must question whether these skills are appropriate for other midwives.

(1) Burnard and Morrison (1991) indicate the difficulty of using a reflective, client-centred approach in the clinical setting.
(2) Much of the work already mentioned emphasises the *structured* nature of the counselling relationship which may conflict with the less than structured clinical workload.
(3) Counselling is not possible while the bereaved person is still in 'a state of numbness or shock', so counselling is unlikely to begin until about a week after the funeral (Worden 1992:39).

Although bereavement counselling may not be appropriate during the few hours or days that the grieving mother spends with us in the maternity area, the approaches and skills used in counselling are certainly likely to be helpful. Using the hospital-orientated approach prevalent in the USA, Davis *et al.* (1988) describe the emotional support which is offered on a less than ideal short-term basis. These authors list some helpful practical interventions:

(1) encouraging acknowledgement of the birth and death of the baby
(2) validating feelings of loss and despair
(3) educating about grief
(4) giving information about choices available

Davis *et al.* go on to consider how staff are able to meet the mother's emotional needs. It is essential to cope with the inevitable feelings of failure among staff, which we must acknowledge to be able to help the mother. Taking time to listen to the mother's sad and angry outbursts shows her that these feelings are acceptable and that her isolation is not complete. Anger directed at staff, us or our colleagues may be difficult to accept, but defensiveness may be defused by remembering that her anger is unfocused rather than specific.

Our fear of not knowing what to say may make us anxious when in this mother's presence, but remembering the value of listening may reduce anxiety. Many writers list unhelpful comments, such as 'You can always have another' and 'I know how you feel', which are best avoided (Davis *et al.*, 1988; Lendrum & Syme, 1992). Opening conversation by saying how we feel about her loss shows her that the knowledge is shared and gives her permission to discuss it.

In a UK setting Kohner and Henley (1992) emphasise the importance of the care of the bereaved mother in the community. The value of the midwife's visits go far beyond the assessment of the mother's physical condition and provide another opportunity for her to ask questions and talk about her loss. Through a detailed knowledge of the location in which she practises, the midwife should also be able to help the mother to make contact with a self-help group. Because the surviving child or children are likely to be around when she visits, the midwife is also able to help the parents support their adjustment.

Summary and discussion

A problem raised by the informants in my recent study which is hardly mentioned in the literature on counselling is the extent to which other staff and possibly the mother may 'miss out' if the counselling role is assumed by one person:

> *Ruby* I don't know if there should be someone specifically in the unit, to help give these mums guidance. I think it's something we've all got to learn to do . . . if you designate one person, you will be left with that person and no one else would bother with them.
>
> *Nancy* They're all counselled, the trouble is that it seems to me that most of them are counselled by nursing officers. They do the actual arrangements or speaking to them, counselling the choices about what they intend to do with the baby, whether they want the hospital to bury the baby or whether they want to make their own funeral arrangements.

The risk of misgivings among other staff is mentioned by Druery (1992) in her role as a bereavement support midwife. She avoids confrontation by not usurping other midwives' roles, offering only support and advice to the midwife and by guiding less-experienced practitioners through the paperwork.

Although the structured approach to counselling which I have described here may have limited relevance to the midwife, the importance of counselling skills in her practice becomes apparent when we consider her twenty-four hour presence. Davis *et al.* (1988) emphasise that we must be available to be with the mother when she feels she is ready to talk. Unlike the counselling model, this may not be at a predetermined time, but may be in the small hours when she is at her lowest ebb and other staff are off duty. It is at this time that the midwife is able to listen and use her 'way of being' to help and support the mother. Although Worden (1992) indicates that the time when midwives are in contact with the mother may be too early for counselling, midwives are ideally suited to help the mother to recognise and accept her feelings before her counselling (if any) begins.

The role of the bereavement counsellor in the maternity area may be questioned, but her existence is invaluable in at least two settings. The first is when grieving has been identified as likely to become pathological such as where the mother lacks support from her family and friends and where her relationship with her partner is poor (Forrest *et al.*, 1982). The second important contribution of the bereavement counsellor is her input into the introduction of students and midwives to death education (Cook & Oltjenbruns, 1989).

In this chapter I have considered what bereavement counselling involves, its place in the maternity area and the extent to which it is appropriate for use by midwives. The role of the counsellor has been shown to be similar to that of the midwife, in that the midwife is 'with woman' through her experience of childbearing, while the counsellor uses her 'way of being' to help resolve grief. For this reason midwives are in the ideal position to offer this form of care.

Chapter 6
Family Grief

When contemplating the effects of grief on a family, the concept of 'Gestalt' is helpful. Defined as 'the whole is greater than the sum of the parts' (Drever, 1964), in this context Gestalt implies both the extent and the interdependence of the components. Family interdependence may not always be easily apparent and as a result the diverse effects of an event, such as a loss, may not be obvious. However, because individual family members are affected by loss, the family system is affected and all members are affected; but through the interaction of the members and their frequent adjustment and readjustment of roles, family homeostasis is usually maintained.

Having noted the integrity of the family system, to examine the differing perceptions and effects of loss I find myself having to separate out the various family members. As far as possible in thinking about family grief, I focus on the effects of perinatal loss, but where specifically relevant authoritative literature is lacking I draw on more general material, such as that relating to the loss of someone older.

Family reactions

The family

The term 'family' is open to a variety of interpretations, depending largely on the cultural context. All too often in the UK the term is used synonymously with 'nuclear family', but I use it in its widest sense to include not only those related through blood and marriage/cohabitation, but also foster, adoptive and step-relations. I include also those less formal adult relations who in the past have been (and sometimes still are) honoured with the title 'uncle' or 'aunt' (Baggaley, 1993).

The family as a system

In order to understand the effects of loss on the family, systems theory is useful because it assists our conceptualisation of family functioning (Cook & Oltjenbruns, 1989; Whyte, 1989).

Systems theory defines the family, first, in terms of being a unit whose interacting parts operate within certain definite boundaries, such as biological and social relationships. Second, the interaction of the members is characterised by varying degrees of openness in communication; a family system which adopts a more closed communicative style is typically less flexible to changes in the external environment as well as being less sensitive to the needs of individual members. Third, as well as physical and other boundaries, the family system operates within its own framework of rules, which may be implicit or explicit. This framework serves to determine the roles of family members within the family system and to maintain, through constant readjustment and realignment, homeostasis of the system. Clearly, family equilibrium or homeostasis is seriously threatened by the death of one of its members.

The degree of threat varies according to features of both the family and the death (Herz, 1980). The threat of disruption depends on, first, the timing of the death in the family life cycle, second, the nature of the death, third, the degree of openness within the family and, fourth, the role of the dead family member.

The re-establishment of family equilibrium will follow realignment of roles and responsibilities. This realignment constitutes a threat both to family stability, and to those most closely involved because at this time they are vulnerable and in a weak position. The factors which inhibit family coping are categorised by Cook and Oltjenbruns (1989); there may be situational stressors, such as unemployment, which may be cumulative, the effects of which are moderated by the strength of family resources. Family coping may be further facilitated by the family's interpretation of the event, in that finding a meaning for the loss renders it more manageable.

Communication within the family

There is a tendency for more responsible members of the family to 'protect' others from the effects of an unpleasant event by limiting communication (Rando, 1986b). We are warned of the danger both to the protectors, who may not allow themselves to grieve appropriately, and to the protected, who are prevented from experiencing a healthy mourning. Rando tells us how parents may seek to protect their surviving children in this way, to the benefit of no-one.

The degree of openness of communication within the system is a family characteristic which affects their ability to grieve a lost child (Stephenson, 1986). Denial of the loss may feature prominently. Stephenson suggests that the closed family behaves in 'bizarre' ways which have been learned from earlier, but possibly dissimilar, experiences. Thus, the inability of this family to accept and share new influences and experiences limits its coping.

The 'conspiracy of silence' which may develop in families following the death of a child is attributed by McNeil (1986) to family guilt. The guilt-ridden and unrealistic beliefs about individual personal responsibility for the death are common to all family members, united only in their inability to share their pain. McNeil (1986) shows us how in these circumstances communication with grief-stricken family members may be assisted by the use of sight, hearing and touch, rather than relying on words.

Communication in a hospice setting was the focus of a research project by Lugton (1989). She drew on Glaser and Strauss' account (1965) of open and closed awareness among dying people and those close to them. Their original research showed the ease of communication when open awareness operated and all involved knew the terminal nature of the illness. In closed awareness, those involved were unable to admit the significance of the illness.

Lugton identified a continuum of degrees of communication between open and closed awareness in her study. Although her interviewees showed understanding of the prognosis, the extent to which this understanding was shared within the family varied hugely. Those families in which awareness was open were able to negotiate new roles during the illness, thus preparing themselves for the subsequent major reallocation of roles. Lugton shows the disquiet within families where closed awareness operated.

Expectations and perceptions

After looking at the social support of widows, Gorer (1965) concluded that the perception of a deficit between expected and actual support impedes grieving. Since then, unhelpful interactions have been implicated as responsible for impeding grieving, on the grounds that grieving widows who reported few or no unhelpful interactions adjusted well. The reverse was true for those widows who perceived more frequent unhelpful activities. The accuracy of these widows' perceptions and the reality of their expectations may be questioned, but we must accept that the perception of unhelpfulness impairs grieving.

In her study, Littlewood (1992) identified four perceived unhelpful factors which operated in this way to impede grieving:

- lack of availability of/access to support
- family disputes over who is the chief mourner
- non-acknowledgement of the relationship between the dead person and the bereaved person
- uncertain social position of the helper.

Parents mourning the loss of a baby may find themselves similarly disappointed by those close to them. They grieve for the baby in whom they had invested hopes and expectations and whom they were coming to know. That their close family are unable to share their loss because they have not been privy to their fantasies may deprive the parents of the anticipated support. Clearly, this discrepancy between expectations and perceptions may lead to conflict.

Fathers

Much of what we know about mothers' grieving applies equally to fathers, but they have some particular problems relating to society's expectations of them and, perhaps, to their expectations of themselves.

Recognising the father's grief

Because his grief is likely to be expressed differently (see below) and because he has not been pregnant, the people who would ordinarily offer support may forget that the father is grieving. Thus, fathers are likely to be deprived of the support which is forthcoming for the mother of the dead baby. The heartfelt plea of a bereaved father is that they 'need to be treated as fathers who have just lost a baby, not as men whose womenfolk are a bit unwell just now' (Fairbairn, 1992).

Writing in the context of miscarriage, but raising issues relevant to other perinatal losses, Raphael-Leff (1991) likens the father's grief to the mother's, but without the social acknowledgement and opportunities for expression. As well as the sense of his childbearing being at the mercy of her body, he also has to cope with not having any tangible bodily changes. These profound feelings may result in the jealousy or ambivalence which he may have initially felt aggravating the guilt of his bereavement (Lewis & Page, 1978).

Male grieving

Kohner and Henley (1992) attribute the reasons why men and women grieve differently to their differing experiences. The physical experience differs, as do expectations and self-image. These authors remind us that western society does not allow men to express their grief through tears.

The difficulty of men crying is discussed by Schatz (1986) using both his experience as a bereaved father and as the organiser of a self-help group. He describes the value of a 'catalyst' such as a photograph or other object in initiating crying and then the fear that, once begun, the tears may never stop. The extent to which the father is able to share or even report his tears varies. Schatz was clearly amazed at the therapeutic value of tears and realises that there are few effective alternatives. The reluctance of fathers to cry was mentioned by mid-wives in my recent research:

Ginnie   ... the partner, you've got to try and remember them too as 'I've got to try and be ever so brave and not cry' or 'I'm a man and I shouldn't be crying...' But they've got to grieve too.

In her study of family networks' influence on bereavement, Kowalski (1987) interviewed five fathers about their experience; they were all surprised by their tearful response. These men felt they carried the burden of making arrangements without really being involved as, like Fairbairn (1992), all the concern is for the mother. They reported that the tears came when they were alone, often driving home or after others were asleep. The fathers felt unable to share their feelings even with the mother, because of their need to protect her. Kowalski concludes that support for grieving men is minimal if not non-existent.

In the same way as expressing emotion has been shown to be more difficult for men, communication is also problematical. Schatz (1986) emphasises the need for men to explain their feelings to other family members, or possibly a self-help group. Implicitly acknowledging the threat of such self-revelation, Schatz suggests a personal journal as an alternative, which carries the advantage of providing feedback by showing how grieving is progressing.

This typically male pattern of grieving was shown by Dyregrov (1991) to be established in boys as early as school age. He found that boys were less able to acknowledge grief and crisis reactions to the sudden death of a teacher. Of particular concern was the inability of boys to express their feelings even in writing, whereas their girl classmates were able to write about their reactions and the benefits of certain interventions. Dyregrov goes on to show how the girls in his sample were better able to locate and confide in a support person, both at home and school. He fails to recognise the greater maturity of girls at the same chronological age, but attributes these differences to the tendency of girls to play more expressively and in pairs, whereas boys prefer competitive, disciplined group activities.

Dyregrov goes on to speculate that males learn at an early age to suppress their feelings in the face of danger, whereas girls learn to confront complex feelings. He argues that the interventions which are provided to support the bereaved are designed more for women's more open style of grieving, leaving men less well-supported in their grief. The midwives told me of their strategies for helping men to begin grieving:

Josie   I give them time to be together for a short time to grieve together especially men – they're not showing their feelings, so I think it's quite nice to just leave them together for a wee while so they can. You find normally that it's the woman that's very upset and everything else, it's the man that's very good and puts a brave face on it for most of the time.

Supporting 'the womenfolk'

Like Dyregrov (1991) Schatz (1986) argues that men learn their stereotypical roles when young. He lists male attributes which may be valued in western society and which conflict with grieving. These are being:

- strong, macho and in control of his emotions
- a winner
- the protector of family and property
- the family provider
- the problem solver – the fixer
- in control of actions and the environment
- self-sufficient and independent.

Schatz compares these roles with the vulnerability and powerlessness characteristic of grieving and demonstrates the incompatibility of these expectations with grief. The result is that the man striving to achieve this style of manhood does not allow himself to grieve. His inability to solve the mother's grief reminds him of his impotence to help and confirms him in his need to appear powerful. He uses up his emotional reserves in maintaining this facade and controlling painful emotions. Eventually his emotions cease to be controlled and escape in angry outbursts at those he least wants to hurt. In a UK culture Long (1992) also observes the counterproductive nature of masculine reactions: 'cultural reserve can get in the way of resolving his own grief'.

The role of the father in supporting the mother of a dying baby is particularly important (Jacques *et al.*, 1983). A study of parental visiting in an NNU showed that the mothers were found to depend heavily on the fathers accompanying them when visiting their newborns. The fathers reported feeling less uncomfortable with and intimidated by the high-tech NNU atmosphere. These researchers further indicate that, far from the damaging role already suggested, this role is actually helpful to the father in establishing new family relationships.

Employment

Men may perceive work as beneficial to grieving, as found during a longitudinal study of 50 bereaved families (Forrest *et al.*, 1983); the coping mechanism widely used by fathers comprised 'plunging them-selves back into work activities'. On the basis of this observation they conclude that fathers have shorter bereavement reactions than mothers.

Kennell and Klaus (1982) discuss the disadvantages of this 'worka-holic' tendency in bereaved fathers. Taking on additional employment and extra community responsibilities means not only that he has no time to confront his feelings, which may be intentional, but he also has no opportunity to share those feelings with those he is close to, especially the mother of their baby.

Endorsing this impression of the grieving father immersing himself in his work, Kowalski (1987) found that most of the fathers she inter-viewed had returned to work within one week of their perinatal loss. These fathers were convinced of the therapeutic value of work, although its value may comprise little more than a temporary distraction from their grief, as Schatz (1986) indicates when he includes excessive overtime as a typically male coping mechanism, along with alcohol and other drugs. He goes on to consider such dysfunctional coping mechanisms' effects on the couple's relationship.

Couples

We tend to assume that babies are always born into relationships like those which we knew as children and which involve people of opposite sexes. This is not necessarily so. In this section particularly we must bear in mind that, though I tend to refer to heterosexual couples because they have been studied, my observations apply equally to lesbian couples. Similarly, my focus on couples should not exclude the unsupported mother who may need to grieve not only the loss of her baby, but also the loss of her relationship with her baby's father.

I have shown in the last section that grief in a man has certain typical characteristics and that the assumption mentioned by Cook and Oltjenbruns (1989) that we all grieve similarly, is invalid. Having looked at men in general, I would now like to look at the differences which have been shown to exist between a couple grieving their baby and at what happens within that couple's relationship when the differences emerge.

Mother/father differences in grieving

Perhaps because the mother is invariably present at the birth, it is usual to use and accept her view of the experience. Whether this is appro-priate when thinking about fathers' reactions is questionable. For this reason I focus here on research which has deliberately sought a balanced view of the couple's experience.

The research by Benfield *et al.* (1978) involved interviewing 50 couples following the perinatal death of their child (see Chapter 8). Utilising seven items in a questionnaire, the researchers drew up a grief score; these items were sadness, poor appetite, sleeplessness, irritability, being preoccupied with the baby, anger and feeling guilty. A self-rating scale (0–3) was completed with 0 indicating 'never a problem' and 3 indicating a major problem. Thus each parent's grief score could range from 0 to 21.

A graph illustrating the couples' grief scores clearly shows the tendency for the mother to have a higher score; this impression is supported by the mothers' mean score (13.4) which significantly exceeded the fathers' mean score (9.7). Although with 10 fathers (20%) his score exceeded hers, this was balanced at the opposite extreme by two fathers who denied any grief. These researchers supported the earlier observation that significantly more mothers experienced episodes of tears. The greater number of mothers feeling guilty was also significant. Fathers' instrumentality is reflected in the observation that, in couples where the father's grief score was high, the couple attended sooner for counselling and discussion of postmortem results.

While Benfield *et al.* suggest that the father's response is less severe, Forrest *et al.* (1983) found that fathers' grieving was of shorter duration than mothers'. They found that 86% of the fathers had recovered from their psychological symptoms within six months, whereas this applied to only 50% of the mothers.

The interpretation of these findings is not completely straightforward. This is partly because of the finding by Kennell *et al.* (1970), on the basis of incomplete and less reliable data, of the fathers' tendency to deny grief. This conflicted with Benfield's observation that they grieved for as long as or longer than the mothers.

Benfield *et al.* (1978) discuss whether the lower grief scores which they found among fathers were due to them having completed their grieving earlier, such as while arranging the funeral and answering enquiries. The researchers' alternative explanation is that the fathers have been prevented from grieving by the burden of responsibility imposed on them and that their delayed grieving has yet to materialise.

An additional reason for the difficulty in interpreting the material on fathers' grieving (Littlewood, 1992), is that men may under-report or fail to acknowledge the disruption which they experience. As Dyregrov (1991) states in the context of young boys, the difficulty which they encounter in articulating their grief may continue into adult life as difficulty in even recognising its existence.

'Dissynchrony' and asymmetry

> *Josie*   It may take them a wee while to accept it, you may have one partner accepting it and the other one not.

Midwife Josie (above) recognised the variation in grieving. The reason why grieving and coping styles assume such significance in the context of perinatal death is associated with the incorrect assumption, mentioned already, that we all grieve similarly. Unfortunately, each parent may assume that, because they have lost the same baby, their grief will manifest itself similarly. They may have difficulty in realising that their coping mechanisms, their hopes and expectations for their baby and their relationship with that baby may not have been identical.

In two parents of different sexes the grieving of each is likely to progress in different ways and at different rates. Each parent may assume that because their partner is not grieving as they are, then they are not grieving at all. Typically, the mother is still overtly grieving while the father is returning to work.

The differences in grieving may be in terms of:

(1) dissimilar gender-determined patterns
(2) 'dissynchrony', meaning that their emotional roller-coasters are poorly aligned
(3) asymmetry or incompatibility in their responses (Rando, 1986b).

With two parents in a highly sensitive and vulnerable state the potential for conflict is massive. One may blame the other for being uncaring while the other makes accusations of wallowing in grief. Each may be unable or unwilling to appreciate the other's viewpoint, if it has been articulated. Each may wonder whether the other's loving feelings towards them have changed. They may feel that they are alone in their grief. In the absence of effective communication each partner will continue to think badly of the other. A form of communication with which the couple may have particular difficulty is their sexual relationship (see Chapter 12).

Changes in the relationship

Inevitably, as the two individuals who make up the couple will be changed by their experience of loss, so their relationship will undergo changes. The effects on the relationship of these changes is a source of contention as serious adverse consequences in the form of breakup have been attributed (Schatz, 1986:296; Kohner & Henley, 1992; Long, 1992; Cook & Oltjenbruns, 1989). Despite reports of a high divorce rate among bereaved parents, no supporting evidence that the breakup is due solely to the loss of a child has been located.

Kowalski (1987) recounts the changing relationship following perinatal loss. She describes the brief and romantic period of supreme closeness following their loss as the 'honeymoon period'. Unfortunately, a deterioration in their relationship follows this initial 'high', which was also observed by Dyregrov and Matthieson (1987) who found increasing strain within the relationship, possibly engendering adverse effects on surviving children.

The impression of an increase in breakups after bereavement is attributed to research ignoring general divorce rates (Rando, 1986b). However, couples with children dying of cancer found that their experience reinforces their relationship by making them more aware of their partner's strengths as opposed to their weaknesses (Foster *et al.*, 1981).

In the event of the relationship becoming difficult following the loss of a baby, Rando (1986b) shows us how secondary losses, for example the loss of family unity, may follow the death which constituted the primary loss. The secondary losses may be real as in this example, or they may be symbolic, such as the lowering of self-esteem. As well as secondary losses, it is not impossible that some secondary gains, such as increased self-knowledge, may eventually present themselves.

Grandparents

The limited research attention given to grandparents and great-grandparents is now beginning to be corrected. According to Smith (1991b) this development is due to demographic changes which mean that grandparents are relatively young and healthy and also due to the increasing fragility of 'marital' relationships, requiring greater contributions from supporting family.

Recognition of the benefits of grandparental involvement in child-rearing is also comparatively recent, which may be associated with demographic changes as well as the modification of ageist attitudes. Their involvement may comprise emotional or financial support or information-giving.

The input of grandparents into childrearing varies according to whether they are maternal or paternal family and grandmothers or grandfathers; maternal grandmothers are most likely to be involved (Smith, 1991b). Additional factors which affect grandparental involvement relate to age, employment, social class, geographical location, ethnic origin, institutionalisation, whether blood relations, and personality (Hurme, 1991).

In the same way as the fathers' role is sometimes assumed to be only to support the mother, the grandparents may be perceived as having no involvement in the process of loss other than to support the parents (McHaffie, 1991). Recent literature does not bear this out.

Loss of future

The significance of the new baby to the grandparents derives from the baby's symbolic representation of the future, and if the baby is lost they perceive a threat to the continuity of the family and life generally (Long, 1992; Rando, 1986b). In certain ways, grandparents consider that because they have invested their hopes and expectations in this baby, the baby belongs to them as well as to the parents (Hurme, 1991). Thus, their grief is increased.

Inability to help their own child

An inability to compensate their children for the loss of their baby or to protect them from grief is a source of misery to grandparents (Borg & Lasker, 1982). Now that they have proved themselves adult in the most obvious way, grandparents are no longer able to fulfil the parental role and feel they have become marginalised and superfluous. Grandparents may underestimate the value of the emotional support they give at difficult times (Smith, 1991b; Tudehope *et al.*, 1986; Kowalski, 1987; McHaffie, 1991).

Survivor guilt

The untimeliness of perinatal death reminds grandparents that as they are nearer the end of their life span it is they, not the new baby, who should die (Borg & Lasker, 1982). The grandparents' grief is compounded by the feeling of inappropriateness of the loss of the young, when the old remain.

Grandparents grieving

In her study of family support and bereavement, Kowalski (1987) interviewed grandparents in five families. In the same way as I noted the reluctance of fathers to cry, the grandfathers were factual and unemotional, whereas the grandmothers were more open in sharing their emotions. The maternal grandmothers' primary concern was the welfare of their daughters; grief at the loss of their grandchild was secondary and paternal grandparents were less involved. As mentioned above, grandparents regretted being unable to protect their child from grief, but failed to relate such feelings to the parents' being bereaved.

The reality of the dead baby was hard for grandparents to accept. Kowalski found that the grief of some of the grandmothers related not to the recently lost baby, but to other losses, earlier in their lives.

The difficulty of grandmothers grieving was also identified in the research by Smialek (1978) on families bereaved through SIDS. The only grandmothers who grieved were those who had been the primary caregiver of the dead child, when profound grief seemed appropriate. Like Kowalski, Smialek found that in other grandmothers their significant grief related to the loss of another, somewhere in the past. Smialek argues that we should provide support for those who grieve, regardless of the source of their grief, and not assume that their sorrow relates only to the current loss.

Loss in multiple pregnancy

The demands and joys of twins are many, especially if the conception follows a period of infertility (Raphael-Leff, 1991). The loss of a twin, or one or more of the babies in a higher multiple birth, has some aspects in common with loss of a singleton, but there are additional potential difficulties.

Gratitude

The assumption may be made that the parents should be so grateful to have one healthy baby that they should not need to grieve the loss of the one who died (Sandbank, 1988). This assumption may hinder the parents' grieving.

Research by Wilson *et al.* (1982) involved a sample of sixteen couples, half of whom had had a singleton baby die perinatally and half of whom had had twins of whom one had died perinatally. Data on the circumstances of the death and the parents' reactions were collected by a three-part questionnaire. The grief of the twins' parents was neither qualitatively nor quantitatively different from the grief of the singletons' parents. Thus, the presence of the living twin in no way ameliorates the impact of their loss. These researchers suggest that, rather than having an easier time, the parents of twins when one dies may actually find more difficulty in grieving for one baby and forming a relationship with another simultaneously.

The problem of grieving one baby

The danger of not grieving the loss of one twin lies in the inevitable eventual manifestation of the grief, possibly in a severely pathological form (Lewis & Page, 1978). The difficulty of grieving one baby and simultaneously beginning a new relationship with another is discussed in Chapter 12.

Lewis and Bryan (1988) discuss the parents' problems of coping with these contradictory psychological processes simultaneously. There is the danger that the dead baby may be dismissed as a mere fantasy; but this can only be a temporary dismissal, with the grieving being nothing more than delayed, appearing later as one of the pathological syndromes of failed mourning. Lewis and Bryan suggest that these pathological outcomes may be avoided by ensuring that the family have experienced the reality of the dead baby, and that they have some tangible memories of it.

Blaming the survivor

The family may show their grief at the loss of a twin by blaming the one who survived (Sandbank, 1988). While blaming the survivor, the dead twin may be idealised; Lewis and Bryan state that this 'angel baby' is particularly likely to materialise if the survivor is in any way unwell or badly-behaved. To make amends, the family may try to compensate by overindulging the baby.

The lone twin

Regardless of whether the other twin dies during pregnancy, infancy or adulthood, the survivor feels some level of responsibility, constituting a form of the survivor guilt mentioned already (Sandbank, 1988). This may be like the separation anxiety seen in older twins.

The difficulty of distinguishing self and not-self in infants may persist in twins and causes problems when a twin does not survive. Sandbank suggests that the parents should be open with the survivor about the death of the twin and be prepared to produce photographs of the babies together to establish their separate identities. The possibility of a child seeking a replacement twin may be avoided by distinguishing them from an early age (Zazzo, 1960 in Sandbank, 1988; Wilson *et al.*, 1982). The dangers of the replacement twin are comparable with the replacement child (see Chapter 12).

The vanishing twin

With the increasing use of ultrasound early in pregnancy, there is increasing awareness of the 'vanishing twin' (Jeanty & Romero, 1984). Possibly because of placental malfunction, one twin does not survive the early months of pregnancy and is reabsorbed or may be found after the birth as a fetus papyraceous. Up to 50% of twin pregnancies end as a singleton birth for this reason (Lewis & Bryan, 1988). Whether to inform the parents of the presence of two babies is a contentious issue, but Bryan (1992) suggests that the family's awareness and grieving of the twin is important.

Sibling perinatal loss

When a child's unborn or newborn sibling dies, the child faces personal disappointment, parental sorrow and general disturbance. As the child grows older and their understanding changes and increases, the meaning of the death also changes from the initial, perhaps guilt-ridden, reaction. Sorrow among parents and other adults means that the child's interpretation of the loss and its current and future significance may be neglected. The consequences for family well-being are far-reaching, but with appropriate care, harm may be avoided.

Our role when caring for bereaved parents is not only to help them to grieve for the one who is lost, but also, and perhaps more challenging, to help them to think of the future for themselves and their family. The care of surviving children is a crucial aspect of our care.

In thinking about sibling reactions to perinatal loss, my focus is primarily on *young* children, particularly of pre-school age. This is because families currently have short age gaps, so it is young children who are more likely to be affected by perinatal sibling loss. The lack of relevant research-based material (Dyregrov, 1988) requires me to use material about other age groups and a case-study (given at the end of this chapter).

Children's understanding

Although children are frequently exposed to death, it is almost invariably through television. This medium detaches the viewer from the reality of the event and does not help a child understand this difficult concept; additionally, viewing the same actor in another programme subsequently may carry false messages. So how does a child learn the meaning of death?

It is usual to think of a child's understanding of death in terms of the developmental stage which they have achieved. The cognitive framework introduced by Piaget is appropriate, envisaging the child passing through stages featuring concreteness, centration, egocentrism, irreversibility, animism and fantasy to reach transductive reasoning (Cook & Oltjenbruns, 1989). In small children concrete thinking predominates and abstractions may be less than helpful, as a midwife told me:

> *Nancy*   a woman who'd had five miscarriages, her first baby was born alive and he was nine . . . and he asked if he could see his brothers and sisters because they had been born here but couldn't come home, so he wanted to see them.

The information given to this boy had not taken account of his understanding. Characteristics of death which we all have ultimately to master are non-functionality, universality, causality and personification. Leon (1990) argues that Piaget's framework (1952) may be less than appropriate for assessing a child's understanding, because there may be factors which prevent a child from articulating these concepts.

Citing Weininger (1979), he recommends that we may gain more valuable insights by observing the child's play. A child's view of life as cyclical may prevent them from accepting that people who die do not come back to life (Dyregrov, 1990). This may be associated with a child's tendency to think in egocentric magical terms, which leads them to think that they can bring the baby back to life; but it may also burden the child with nagging anxieties about their responsibility for the baby's death. A child who initially felt ambivalent about the 'arrival of a rival' (Kayiatos, 1984) may encounter guilt because of their hostile thoughts (Lewis & Page, 1978). Their egocentricity may initiate a guilty circle of non-communication if their parents are unable to provide factual information (McNeil, 1986).

Because a child may not fully comprehend the implications of the word 'death', their reaction to being given sad news may be quite different from that of an older person. They may not accept the permanence of death, as the concept of future time may not yet be real. Such 'inappropriate' and apparently callous reactions may cause pain to a grieving parent.

Raphael-Leff (1991) discusses the difficulties which a child may face, focusing particularly on denial as a way of coping with loss. She suggests that fantasies may become established as part of denial, which serve to retard the grieving process. While we are aware of the fantasies which mothers who have not seen their stillborn babies may harbour, Dyregrov (1988) maintains that the fantasies of uninformed children are yet more fearful (see the case history at the end of this chapter).

The age at which a child's understanding is enough for them to be informed of loss is a contentious point (see the case history at the end of this chapter). It clearly relates to the developmental stages already mentioned; some authors suggest a specific age, such as 18 months (Kuykendall, 1989). It is difficult to imagine that an even younger child is unaware of the disruption and grief among those near to them, and hence deserves appropriate love, care and explanations.

Physical and behavioural responses

An important feature of the ground-breaking research by Dyregrov (1988) was its detailed description of sibling grief in a healthy population. This researcher followed up 75 families who had experienced a perinatal death or early SIDS and had surviving children; there was a 55% response rate to his initial approach. A longitudinal design collected quantitative and qualitative data from parents about the grief of 3–9 year-olds.

Anxiety was found to be a prominent if short-term feature, which was apparent in the child's sleeping difficulties and concern about parental health. The child constantly sought meaning by questioning the why's and how's of the loss. Repetitive questioning allowed the child to obtain new information and integrate it with old. Many questions were of a practical nature, relating to the location of heaven, activities in the grave and nourishment. The child blaming the parents and showing anxiety about poor caretaking disturbed them. The child's angry and aggressive responses indicated an existing affection for the dead child. Although elements of guilt are generally thought to prevail, Dyregrov found little evidence of this.

Behaviourally, Dyregrov identified increasing demands among the grieving children, which were more pronounced in children who had been separated from their parents by being sent to stay with family. Regressive behaviour also features in a child's grief response, including overdependency, separation anxiety, eneuresis and social withdrawal (Cook & Oltjenbruns, 1989)

An issue raised by Dyregrov (1988), which makes the interpretation of his data more difficult, is the close positive correlation between the parental and sibling reactions. The impact of parental grief causes the child to become confused and fearful. The difficulty of separating the child's reaction to the death from the child's reaction to parental grief is aggravated by the tendency of a young child to imitate parental behaviour (Elizur & Kauffman, 1983; see also the case history at the end of this chapter). The absence of direct or observational data about the children compound this problem.

Interventions

On the basis of his research, Dyregrov (1988) recommends that the care of grieving children should focus on four areas which I will now discuss.

Open and honest communication

The child should be given an explanation appropriate to their under-standing and age, which may be assisted by real-life examples (Kuykendall, 1989) such as the death and burial of a pet or small animal.

In order to reduce the child's confusion euphemisms for death should be strenuously avoided. Although the thesaurus lists many alternative words, a child would find difficulty applying them; others would actually cause greater confusion. Examples are 'laid to rest' or 'gone to sleep', which may engender fear of these activities in a child. Similarly, the commonly-used euphemism 'lost' may cause yet more confusion (Borg & Lasker, 1982).

Although adults may find religious observance a solace in grief, complex religious concepts may perplex a small child (Stephenson, 1986), although one midwife recommended such analogies:

Irene I sometimes tell the mother to tell the other children that the new baby was too good for this world and that it has gone to heaven.

An abstract concept, like heaven, presents problems to a toddler. In order to tell children sad news, there may be difficulty in opening up the topic (see the case history at the end of this chapter). Questions to probe the child's understanding of the situation may achieve both ends (Hardgrove & Warrick, 1974). Dyregrov (1991) recommends that accurate factual information should always be consistently emphasised. Smialek (1978) used this principle to encourage children she counselled to understand the reasons for their siblings' deaths, by correcting guilty misconceptions.

The extent to which children may be made less uncomfortable with their loss, through effective communication, is illustrated by a personal account in which a four year-old caused embarrassment by publicly discussing her dead brother (Beard, 1989).

Parents have traditionally tried to protect their children from pain by not informing them of a loss (see the case history at the end of this chapter). This is merely parental self-protection and in no way benefits the child (Dyregrov, 1988). Ideally, parents should give this information, but, unfortunately, they are temporarily, through their own grief, least able to offer it. However, the expression and sharing of sorrow may benefit both parent and child, as when children comfort their grieving parents (Dyregrov, 1988; Beard, 1989).

Giving time for cognitive mastery

Helping the child's understanding may be time-consuming and painful, but the information needs to be given in packages that the child is able to assimilate. Questioning and openness should be encouraged and may be assisted by more tangible mementoes, such as photographs and items belonging to the baby (see the case history at the end of this chapter).

Visiting the grave is a way of encouraging the child to recognise their loss. Despite cultural opposition to children attending the funeral, Dyregrov found that 35% of his sample had accompanied parents to visit the grave later, although this may have been for convenience. Despite sounding incongruous, children may be encouraged to work through their grief by play (Cook & Oltjenbruns, 1989).

Making the loss real

In the Dyregrov sample almost none of the children had seen their dead sibling, the exceptions being the SIDS deaths. In cultures where viewing the body is usual, children are often exempt, but attitudes to children seeing or even holding the dead baby are changing (Brierley, 1988).

The child needs to be both prepared for this experience and accompanied by a supportive adult (Dyregrov, 1988, 1991).

Adequate preparation and a specific support person are also essential if, after having been given the choice, the child elects to attend the funeral. Although Dyregrov (1988) considers that attendance is likely to help the child, he stresses that no force or encouragement should be applied. Alternative goodbyes may be arranged if the child decides against the funeral, such as special services or other events (Cook & Oltjenbruns, 1989).

Perhaps because it is widely used in the UK and because it raises special issues, cremation needs to be mentioned. Dyregrov (1991) suggests that particularly full explanations are essential, as well as suitable follow-up of the development of understanding. Recognising the loss may also be facilitated by parents showing their own feelings openly and by not hiding away mementoes of the dead baby (see the case history at the end of this chapter).

Stimulating emotional coping
The practice of 'protecting' a child by removing them from their usual surroundings at a difficult time serves only to increase their separation anxiety (Raphael-Leff, 1991; Dyregrov, 1988; see also the case history at the end of this chapter). He found that children who had been separated from their parents became obsessively overprotective towards them.

As well as having a specific adult to accompany a child at sensitive times, Raphael-Leff (1991) recommends that a facilitator should be available to help the child to grieve. In her role as a school nurse Simmons (1992) identifies her contribution.

Summary

This chapter has examined some of the wider-ranging effects of perinatal loss. The diversity of the family and the multiplicity of inputs increases the family's strength and ability to withstand the onslaughts to which it is vulnerable. Despite this, it is apparent that difficulties may arise within families at this time, perhaps associated with all family members being affected, albeit in differing ways, by the death. The extent of threat posed by these difficulties relates to the openness of family communication.

A case history

When I met her she had difficulty recalling the details. She had only been about 10 at the time. It had happened almost 40 years earlier. She thought then that she knew about babies:

I'd been around when mummy had my younger brother – so I knew all about it!

During the winter she helped her mother to prepare for the forthcoming birth:

> We got the cot out. Mummy knitted vests. We cleaned her bedroom so that it would be OK for when the midwife came. Everybody said how good I was – 'A proper little midwife' they all said. (She laughed wryly.)

She felt surprised and confused when nothing happened – there was no new baby. She knew that when someone was going to have a baby, they had a baby:

> But mummy didn't.

She recalled her mother having to stay in bed, but didn't know why. Then things began to disappear: the cot was put away and the knitting stopped. She was aware of people round about being very kind to her:

> But nobody told me what was happening. It was obvious I wasn't meant to ask. So I didn't. They probably thought I'd forgotten about the baby. When pancake day came round, we were sent to the doctor's house for our dinner. It was meant to be a treat. I was sent away to stay with my aunt for Easter.

Some time later she was amazed when her father called in to see her at school.

> He never usually set foot in the place. He sat on the steps and gave me a new wind-cheater he'd brought for me. I couldn't understand why.

After school that day her older sister, who was a student nurse, took her shopping. One of the shopkeepers enquired after their mother:

> My sister said she'd had a boy, but that he was born dead. Because I wasn't meant to talk about it, I didn't say anything.

She believes that the reason nobody said anything to her about the baby's death was that they thought her too young to understand. Shortly before her father died, he told her of his sorrow at losing that baby.

She still thinks of the baby and to her he is Michael. She still finds herself wondering what Michael was like and whether he was properly formed. She wonders if he is buried somewhere, or what happened to him.

She believes that although she has never been told anything about him, she learned a lot from Michael. She learned that there are some things that you just do not talk about, but for a long time she was unsure why.

Was it because it doesn't matter when someone dies? To her it looked like that because nobody seemed to bother and nobody cried.

Or was it because dying is too awful to speak about? She has since learned that some things are better talked about.

Or was it that babies don't matter? In a big family like hers, she wondered whether one child mattered.

Perhaps she had been told about it – when the shopkeeper was:

> I think I was being protected by not being told directly. I'm sure they thought it was best.

Chapter 7
Bereavement and HIV/AIDS

Bereavement may dominate the life of a woman with human immuno-deficiency virus (HIV)/acquired immune deficiency syndrome (AIDS). This is partly because of her own death having been brought unexpectedly closer and partly because of the deaths of friends, lovers and, perhaps, children. Currently, we believe that a foreshortened life span faces most people with HIV infection (Sherr, 1989a).

We must handle data on HIV/AIDS with care, because it is an area in which research and, hence, knowledge is far from complete. Our knowledge about HIV/AIDS is growing day by day and much of what we believed to be factually correct in the early 1980s when these conditions were relatively new, has since been questioned. Examples include the effects of pregnancy on the progression of HIV to AIDS (Brettle & Leen, 1991) and the likelihood of vertical transmission (European Collaborative Study, 1991).

To further justify my cautious approach, there are many reasons why statistical information may be less than accurate, including 'logistic, social and even political reasons' (Kay, 1989). Kay, like Morlat *et al.* (1992), suggests that statistics underestimate the number of women affected and that globally the number of AIDS cases and AIDS-related deaths may be twice the reported figure.

In this chapter, however, I intend to focus more on the *issues* relating to bereavement and death associated with HIV/AIDS than on epidemiological statistics and clinical 'facts'. I begin by taking a wide-ranging view of the development of these conditions. I then focus on women and HIV/AIDS, their sexual behaviour and the associated childbearing issues. This will bring me round to thinking specifically about death and bereavement and the help available to those who have to cope with AIDS-related deaths. I then move on to look at the broader issues which HIV/AIDS and the likelihood of death raise for all of us and particularly for those who care for childbearing women and their families.

Background

The 'silent', that is, unnoticed by health care agencies, spread of HIV infection began during the 1970s. That it is continuing inexorably is evidenced by the number of deaths due to the major effect of this infection, AIDS. Worldwide the virus is spread by the passage of infected body fluids by the same three routes:

- through sexual intercourse
- through the exchange of blood by using contaminated skin-piercing objects
- through 'vertical' transmission from mother to child (Goedert *et al.*, 1991).

The virus may take one of at least two major forms; HIV-2 is prevalent in sub-Saharan Africa. The other form (HIV-1) is primarily responsible for infections throughout the remainder of the world (Kay, 1989). This chapter focuses on HIV-1, henceforth called 'HIV'.

Women's issues

Prior to the mid-1980s the concept of 'high risk' groups included gay men, intravenous drug users (IVDUs) and IVDUs' sexual partners (Bury, 1992). The recognition of the increasing spread of HIV into the female heterosexual population in the mid-1980s rendered the concept of 'high risk' groups redundant (Norman *et al.*, 1990); the focus of concern moved to 'high risk' *behaviour* (Sherr & George, 1989). At that point HIV/AIDS ceased to be only a problem of minority groups, but became a universal concern.

The factors which affect the progression of HIV infection to AIDS have been widely studied in men and in IVDUs, but the ways in which the disease progresses in women, and particularly in those outside the childbearing population, have been largely underresearched (Brettle & Leen, 1991; Robertson *et al.*, 1990).

Prognosis
The prognosis for women who are HIV positive, in spite of meagre research, is widely recognised as poorer than for men (Brettle & Leen, 1991; Kell & Barton, 1991; Critchley, 1992). The *reasons* for women's poorer outcomes are less clear. The different health care system in the USA, where much of the research has been done, may account for some of the difference, due to many women being unable to afford health care; but whether these poorer prognoses are due to health care organisation, IVDU, gender, other or a combination of factors remains unclear.

Diagnosis
Difficulties inherent in making the diagnosis may account for the poorer prognosis for women (Critchley, 1992). Women's signs and symptoms

tend to be less specific than those presented by men. Examples of women's symptoms include general malaise, genital herpes, candidiasis, vaginal discharge and generalised lymphadenopathy (Kell & Barton, 1991). Although female-specific conditions are found more commonly and are of greater severity in HIV positive women than in other women (Bury, 1992), at the time of writing none are included in the definition of AIDS used by the Communicable Diseases Surveillance Centre. The absence of a clear diagnostic description of HIV/AIDS in women causes many problems, including being ineligible for financial and other benefits which are only available to diagnosed persons with AIDS. Bury (1992) states that 'many women die from HIV-associated conditions without a diagnosis of AIDS and [hence] women are under-represented in AIDS statistics'.

The problem of making the diagnosis in women is compounded by the rarity of one of the early and obvious symptoms. Superficial forms of Kaposi's sarcoma facilitate men diagnosing themselves as HIV positive, because it indicates HIV infection at an early stage. This symptom encourages the man to present himself for screening and possibly care. In Caucasian women, Kaposi's sarcoma is unusual (Morlat *et al.*, 1992), so this early warning does not operate.

Awareness

The lack of awareness of women with AIDS further reduces the likelihood that a woman's symptoms, such as respiratory tract infection, would be correctly diagnosed; whereas in a man *Pneumocystis carinii* would be diagnosed promptly (Friend, 1992). Thus, the failure to diagnose her condition correctly may result in the woman's death in her first severe illness.

The delay in making the diagnosis may account for women's shorter survival rates, partly because the presenting illness may be fatal and partly because the disease is further advanced at diagnosis, making intervention less appropriate. Like Bury, Morlat *et al.* (1992) plead for medical practitioners to be more aware of the likelihood of HIV-related infections in women.

Women and sexual behaviour

The public outcry, stimulated by ill-informed media, which greeted the early recognition of HIV/AIDS was ineffective in influencing sexual behaviour and limiting the spread of HIV/AIDS. Holland *et al.* (1990) suggest that while judgemental attitudes were focused on 'high risk' groups during the 'gay plague' media hype, complacent denial became established among those outside the then-acknowledged risk categories.

The original adverse media exposure may have been one reason why gay men have been so successful in changing their behaviour towards safer sex (Aggleton & Homans, 1988; Bor, 1990). Unfortunately, the same cannot be said for heterosexual people. The behaviour change which *safer heterosexual sex* requires, particularly involving condom use, carries mixed and confusing messages. (The term 'safer' sex is used in this chapter because even protected sex is not risk-free.) This is due to condoms' traditional and less than totally effective contraceptive function: 'Contraceptives which are most effective in preventing pregnancy are least effective in protecting against STDs [sexually transmitted diseases]' (IPPF, 1991).

The safer sex message's limited impact on heterosexual behaviour is demonstrated in research on young women's attitudes (Holland *et al.*, 1990), which showed the relative powerlessness of women in negotiating the use of condoms for protection against HIV during penetrative sex. Holland *et al.* conclude that women attach not inconsiderable significance to safer sex; but these young women fear that if they assert their decision, their dreams of trust, romance and spontaneity within their sexual relationships will be threatened.

A similar picture is presented by a mature woman working with people with AIDS (Anon, 1990). She observes, without regret, her recent avoidance of one night stands, but acknowledges even *her* difficulty in expecting any future long-term sexual partner to practise safer sex until both have 'negative HIV tests'.

Women working in *the sex industry* have, like gay men, heeded the safer sex message (Fitzpatrick *et al.*, 1989), although their difficulties in implementing such practices are not unlike those of Holland's sample. Anxiety that prostitutes are responsible for spreading HIV (Morlat *et al.*, 1992) seems to have stimulated the development of schemes to increase the education and support available to women prostitutes (Jacques, 1992; Lyall, 1992), and research focusing on condom use among women sex workers emphasises the continuing need for education about safer sex (de Graaf *et al.*, 1993).

Women and childbearing

Despite impressions to the contrary, conception, pregnancy and childbearing are still major side-effects of heterosexual intercourse. It is unsurprising that an infection spread via intercourse should cause concern for both the baby and the mother, although the former tends to predominate (Denenberg, 1992).

Childbearing decision-making

For many women *the decision to become pregnant* is deliberate and conscious. There is no reason to think that this is any different for women with HIV/AIDS. The desire for a child may be more acute in a woman who perceives her own life span as being unnaturally foreshortened. On the other hand, if her view of her condition is more negative, she may consider that she has too little to offer a child, in terms of the quality or duration of care thus seeking to avoid pregnancy. She may then find that childlessness becomes a dreaded prospect. An intermediate stance would be for the woman to delay childbearing while awaiting a cure for HIV/AIDS. Unfortunately, this may not be a realistic option for those whose biological clocks are ticking away.

As pregnancy was at one time thought to accelerate the progression of HIV to AIDS (Lapointe *et al.*, 1985), she may be concerned about speeding up the deterioration in her health. She may be aware of the previously accepted high vertical transmission rate, and be unwilling to expose a child to such a high risk (European Collaborative Study, 1991). She may suspect that because of her HIV status, the health of her baby may be jeopardised in other ways before it is even born (Johnstone *et al.*, 1988). Clearly, the most up-to-date information should be made available to the woman making childbearing decisions.

Whether to continue her pregnancy may pose a dilemma to a woman with HIV who finds herself pregnant. A research project examined the pregnancy-continuation decisions of 'high risk' women; there were 163 pregnancies and 44 women knew that they were HIV positive (Johnstone *et al.*, 1990). These researchers found that the incidence of termination of pregnancy (TOP) was increased threefold in this 'high risk' group compared with other women, but that HIV status was the primary reason for TOP in only a minority of the women. There were clearly many other important events in these women's lives that influenced their decision.

Johnstone *et al.* endorse the limited effect of HIV status by drawing our attention to the stability of the women's decisions, in that the women in this sample did not change their minds about continuing the pregnancy after an HIV test. These researchers argue that these mothers may have had an unrealistically optimistic perception of the effects of HIV/AIDS due to the early stage of the disease in their peers. The researchers warn us that women may decide on TOP more frequently when more seriously ill women become more visible. It remains to be seen whether this condescending prediction proves correct.

HIV testing in pregnancy

Testing antenatally is advocated on epidemiological grounds (Chrystie *et al.*, 1992; Hepburn, 1992; McCarthy *et al.*, 1992), but there is a danger that HIV testing may become just another in the battery of tests used to screen pregnant women (Roth & Brierley, 1990). The likelihood of this happening is increased by the tendency of our medical colleagues to assume that an intervention which benefits a small, well-defined group will inevitably benefit all mothers.

The argument in favour of routine HIV testing in pregnancy hinges on convenience, that is, the availability of large numbers of evidently sexually active women, who are giving specimens of blood anyway. That pregnant women constitute a representative sample is questionable due to their obvious non-practice of safer sex and the increased likelihood of their being in a stable relationship (Sherr, 1991).

The differences between HIV testing and other antenatal screening tests are fundamental (Sherr, 1991).

The *limitations* of HIV testing arise partly from the existence of the twelve week 'window' when the person is infected and infectious, but antibody is unidentifiable (Sherr & George, 1989). The HIV test has no predictive value as to the progress of HIV/AIDS or even the stage of the disease at the time of testing. The test does not predict the effect on the fetus/neonate (McCarthy *et al.*, 1992).

The *psychosocial implications* of the test and of the result for the woman, her baby and those close to her constitute another fundamental difference between this and other antenatal tests. The need for informed consent prior to testing, whether named or anonymous, inevitably requires that effective pre- and post-test counselling must be routinely available (Roth & Brierley, 1990).

The *epidemiological argument* is obviously and inherently flawed. The existence of the 'window' means that data collected in antenatal clinics *must* underestimate the prevalence of HIV/AIDS. The limited validity of any data collected raises ethical questions about this form of epidemiological research.

Further ethical questions arise from considering who *benefits* from testing. The woman and her baby will not benefit because treatment of HIV/AIDS is at a rudimentary stage (Gibb & Newell, 1992). The staff do not benefit, because HIV status does not determine infection control measures (Kennedy & Edwards, 1993). The argument that interventions are inappropriate unless the patient benefits is decisive (Sherr, 1991).

The carers

Informal carers

The informal carers make up an increasingly significant proportion of health care. Reporting on a San Francisco conference, Bor (1990) outlines the complex inputs by considering the family in terms of the biological family and the social family (including lovers/friends). Stigmatisation of an affected family may engender ostracism, which may unite the family.

He also recounts the intergenerational disruptions which affect informal caring, such as the death of affected parents leading to elderly grandparents caring for a dying child. Alternatively, a youngster who may be infected may care for their dying mother. The existence of these informal arrangements are well-established in African countries and are now recognised in the USA (Panos, 1990).

Biological families' disadvantage compared with social families was poignantly recounted by the guilt-ridden father of an infected child: 'families do not have the networks of support to which many people in the gay community have access'.

'Buddys'

The formal/informal care divide has been bridged by a system of care known as 'Buddying' (Veksner, 1993). Begun in the USA, this is now organised in the UK by the Terence Higgins Trust. People with AIDS may seek a 'Buddy', who has volunteered to offer practical and emotional support and friendship. Certain ground rules operate, such as the person with AIDS being able to reject the Buddy, but the Buddy must stay with their contact for at least 12 months. Apart from a ban on sexual contact, Buddying is what the two people make of it.

Health care staff

That health care staff make a significant contribution in the care of women with HIV/AIDS was established by Mok (cited in Bor, 1990). She found that 75% of the HIV positive IVDU women in her sample rated health care staff as their main source of support; this was in preference to even their own biological family.

The relevance of the traditional midwifery role in the care of a mother with AIDS is also clear (Dick, 1992). The midwife is shown to be supporting, advising and 'being with' a mother throughout her experience of childbearing. Despite the satisfactions which undertaking this fundamentally important role brings, it also carries an additional burden of stress which work-related support helps to resolve (Sherr & George, 1988).

The additional stress is due to helping the mother to cope with her anxieties, combined with the risks of infection which maternity care may carry. The irrelevance of HIV testing of mothers to us as carers is emphasised repeatedly in the literature. In the context of infection control, Kennedy and Edwards (1993) show us that knowledge of a mother's serostatus is no substitute for conscientious implementation of the Universal Precautions as protection against infection (Wilson & Breedon, 1990).

Our need to protect ourselves and those we love from infection may arouse 'misguided fears' (Sherr, 1991) perhaps resulting in 'refusal to care' (Jemmott *et al.*, 1992). Likewise, similar fears have arisen among some for whom we care; the anxiety being that infected health care professionals may transmit the virus to 'patients'. Our correct use of the Universal Precautions means inevitably that by effectively protecting ourselves, we protect those for whom we care.

Ill-informed media scares demonstrate that 'misguided fears' are not unique to carers. The need for education to allay such fears and develop more accurate knowledge and appropriate attitudes among health care providers has been established in a series of studies (Bond & Rhodes, 1990; Bond *et al.*, 1990). Perhaps the media are similarly in need of education.

Loss, bereavement and death

Pre-test counselling

The impact of HIV/AIDS begins with the realisation that the HIV test may, for whatever reason, be necessary. During pre-test counselling, the person contemplates why a test is needed and what implications she envisages the result (positive or negative) will have for her and for those she loves. Bor (1991) defines the counsellor's role as providing a suitably secure and comfortable physical and emotional environment in which, with accurate information, the person is able to identify concerns and make decisions.

Post-test counselling

In post-test counselling a negative result requires the person to contemplate avoidance of her 'risky' behaviour which made the test necessary. If the test is positive the person needs the support of the counsellor to cope with her immediate reaction to this information.

The counsellor helps the person with a positive result to anticipate the many losses which she is likely to encounter. Some understanding of the stages in the dying and grieving process may help her to be aware of her own reactions, although we must bear in mind the limitations of using a theoretical framework. In the context of HIV, Sherr (1989a) and George (1992) criticise the existing accounts of grieving as being prescriptive timetables, as they provide no insight into the underlying reasons for the unfolding pattern of grief and no help in planning care.

George's recommendation for more effective counselling combines a systems approach (Jenkins, 1989) with personal construct theory (Bannister & Fransella, 1986).

Systems theory adopts a holistic view of our existence, in which any change carries inevitable repercussions for other interrelated parts. Systems theory is useful in considering the implications for, for example, the biological family when a person with AIDS seeks reconciliation.

The application of personal construct theory recognises the rationality of people, within the limits of their own knowledge. Their rationale allows internally logical decisions and plans, which may not be comprehensible to others. George (1992) suggests that counsellors need to recognise these processes in clients in order to comprehend their attitudes and behaviour and to help them make realistic plans.

Coping with losses

While recognising our difficulty in coping with multiple losses (George, 1992) and, hence, the crucial need for counselling and support, Sherr (1989a) lists the losses which the person with HIV/AIDS faces.

The prospect of loss of *life* immediately springs to mind. Facing up to mortality when a further forty or fifty years of life had been expected means that time is of the essence for this person. Unfinished business will need to be finished off urgently (Catania *et al.*, 1992).

Loss of *health* is second, which includes the general malaise which many of the opportunistic infections carry with them, as well as the more upsetting effects, such as the inexorable itching of vaginal thrush. More debilitating conditions, such as the incapacitating diarrhoea caused by cryptosporidium, carry social as well as physical implications.

Sherr mentions the loss of *relationships* as the third loss. This may mean the loss through death of lovers, friends and family. Sorrow due to the loss of 'friends' because of the stigma of HIV/AIDS may be more real than their friendship was; this is aggravated by the difficulty of establishing a new social network. Prior to becoming infected, relationships with the biological family may have deteriorated for some people with AIDS because of unconventional lifestyles (George, 1992).

The change in or loss of sexual relationships, associated with practising safer sex, carries the loss of a form of human closeness, contact and communication. A woman with HIV infection may find difficulty in making contact with people in a non-sexual way, resulting in isolation. Regret at her need to change sexual practices will be aggravated by her loss of libido, due to declining health.

The loss of *children* may be due to death resulting from the rapid course which HIV/AIDS follows in the very young (European Collaborative Study, 1991). The decision to have children who risk being infected, to have an existing pregnancy terminated or not to have children at all brings the need to mourn the loss of what for many is an all-too-easy process.

A mother's decision about what and when to tell existing, uninfected older children will be determined partly by her guilt and anguish (Barlow, 1992); her relationship with these children will be affected, perhaps damaged, when they are informed of their mother's HIV/AIDS diagnosis.

The threat to her *self-image* may concern the young woman brought up in a society that values highly physical appearance. The change in body contours due to wasting may be perceived negatively, as may alopecia due to cytotoxic drugs used to treat neoplasms.

Economic losses may arise from the stigma carried by HIV/AIDS, causing loss of employment and housing difficulties.

The final loss mentioned by Sherr is the *fear* of losses, such as fear of the loss of clarity of thought in AIDS dementia. These feared losses include the 'dreaded issues', identified as including disfigurement and pain (Perakylaa & Bor, 1990).

In a later work, Sherr (1991) adds the loss of *control* to her list. This lack or loss of control may relate to the concept of 'locus of control', which is the ability to take control of one's life (Wallston & Wallston, 1981). This characteristic is an enduring, personality quality which transcends the immediate situation and includes the expectancy that a person with certain personality characteristics will act in a certain way. Locus of control comprises a person's perception, developed over many experiences, of what causes things to happen in their lives.

The locus of control may be external, when the person tends to blame others or their environment or it may be internal, when the person blames themself or assumes responsibility. A person with an external locus of control really believes that the things that they do cannot influence outcomes.

The converse is someone with an internal locus of control who believes that outcomes are contingent upon their actions. There may be a tendency towards one extreme or the other in that a person may be 'more internal' or 'more external'. For a woman whose personality incorporates an internal locus of control, being required by illness to adopt a more 'external' approach will engender feelings of passivity, or even resignation. As in so many areas, our aim in caring for, as well as counselling, this woman is to encourage her to retain control over the choices which she wants to make (Mander, 1993).

Sherr (1989a) also identifies the feelings of loss of a *future*, making a nonsense of living and engendering an overwhelming sense of futility. This lack of a future presents a major challenge to those affected, to carers and to counsellors. Support to facilitate coping with feelings of futility constitutes a crucial aspect of the care of people with AIDS. This point is emphasised when Sherr discusses other psychological reactions of people with AIDS, such as depression, anxiety, fear and suicidal thoughts. Sherr emphasises the need to take such thoughts seriously if and when they are articulated. The possibility of assisted suicide and euthanasia are discussed by Almond (1990), alongside the ethical issues relating to humane limits of treatment and the right to die.

Support

The support available to and used by people with HIV/AIDS is, for reasons indicated already, dynamic – changing as the disease and our knowledge of it progresses. A prospective research project was undertaken by Catania *et al.* (1992) to trace the support which a sample of 52 gay men sought as their health status deteriorated. To focus on help in coping with death anxiety, the men were categorised according to whether they were HIV positive or not, and whether the HIV positive men were symptomatic.

Overall, lovers and friends were the primary source of support. The men's biological families assumed greater importance as their condition deteriorated, in terms of both help being sought and given. Clearly, barriers which existed earlier in their lives due to estrangement had been overcome. The decreasing input by lovers and friends may be attributed to their relative youth and inexperience about death, or to their own feelings of mortality.

Coping with death

Although we may assume that death itself constitutes a major source of anxiety, Sherr (1991) suggests that it is dying which is more frightening. Hinton (1977) attributed this to fear of uncontrolled and uncontrollable pain, which may not be unreasonable when we consider how rare it is for lay people to witness natural death. Sherr describes her research with George (1989) which showed that for people with AIDS, fear of stigmatisation outweighs fear of pain. This condemnation of society's attitudes towards dying people is magnified by the anxiety being not entirely unjustified (Jemmott *et al.*, 1992).

Discussion

According to Carovano (1991), the problems which women world-wide are likely to encounter as the HIV/AIDS pandemic develops are comparable to those already experienced by women in developing countries (Panos, 1990). She demonstrates the relative powerlessness of women in their sexual relationships and the need for the woman to persuade or cajole her partner into practising safer sex, as the tendency is for a woman to choose contraceptive methods which do not 'inconvenience' her partner.

Carovano goes on to plead for the empowerment of women by the introduction of devices which effectively protect her from infection and which allow her to conceive as and when she wishes. Devices which protect women from HIV while permitting conception become more necessary when we take account of the relative risks of heterosexual intercourse.

Men transmit HIV more effectively, as their transmission rates may be twice that of their women partners (Ward Davies, 1990). More authoritative estimates are considerably higher; an example is found in data collected in New York (Handsfield, 1988) which show that whereas up until August 1987 only 5 men had contracted HIV heterosexually, 263 women had become infected in this way. The risk of contracting HIV, and of dying from AIDS, escalates exponentially if a person happens to be a woman. This is due initially to her inability to insist on safer sex and then to her increased risk of infection when risky sex is practised.

In addition to the woman's risk of infection being increased, her vulnerability to being infected and dying may be being compounded by the lack of research and media attention. Media exposure is essential to overcome the next major hurdle – that of convincing women that the risk message applies to *them* (Carovano, 1991).

The lack of attention given to women and HIV/AIDS has been noted in the nursing media (Bury, 1992; Friend, 1992) and has been utilised more generally (Carovano, 1991; Holland *et al.*, 1990; Critchley, 1992). These authors have commented on the invisibility of women in the context of HIV/AIDS and the way in which the effect of AIDS on women is defined only in terms of their relationships with others. This is clearly apparent in the attention given to women who work in the sex industry and who may be perceived as a 'reservoir' of infection constituting a danger to men (Morlat *et al.*, 1992) rather than as another group of vulnerable people.

The considerable and probably appropriate research attention given to 'vertical transmission' is another example of the neglect of the infection in women (Dunn *et al.*, 1992; Hu *et al.*, 1992; Goedert *et al.*, 1991).

Summary

During its relatively brief history, HIV/AIDS has become synonymous with loss. Initially the deaths were those of gay men and IVDUs. With growing realisation that the virus could be transmitted through heterosexual intercourse, the dangers of spread by women working in the sex industry developed. Perinatal risks and neonatal/infant death next became a serious concern, focusing on 'vertical transmission' and the determining factors. More accurate information of the risks to the baby has allowed attention to turn eventually to other issues; these are the effects on mothers and then on women in general.

Increasing numbers of women's deaths represents the end of a long line of infections. Having been infected by a long-term heterosexual partner (Carovano, 1991), they may have unknowingly infected their children, who may have died more quickly. These losses, together with their own foreshortened life span, may convince mothers of the futility of existence (Sherr, 1989a).

Our role as carers is to help women to avoid becoming infected, but if our intervention is too late, we must support the woman in making and implementing the right choices for her. In the later stages of her infection, we may be able to help her to focus on her living, rather than her dying; ensuring that while the duration of her life may be limited, its quality will not be. In this way she will be able to make the most of what life has to offer; in the words of Brown and Powell Cope (1991) she will be 'maximising the present'.

Chapter 8
Grief in the Neonatal Unit

A baby is admitted to the neonatal unit (NNU) either because a health problem has been recognised or because there is a real possibility of such a problem arising. Regardless of diagnosis, the parents of this baby have to adjust to the likelihood of a condition which threatens health, or even life. In order to make this adjustment the parents must grieve for the ideal baby they expected and have lost (Lancaster, 1981; Moore, 1981; Sherr, 1989b), before being able to relate to the baby who has been born (see Chapter 1). Thus, even in the absence of death, grief features prominently in the NNU.

A further factor requiring adjustment in these parents is the non-fulfillment of the role which they had anticipated. Ordinarily the mother is able to satisfy her baby's everyday needs, and in doing so she is likely to have the support of nurses, midwives and health visitors. For a mother whose baby has been admitted to the NNU, the situation is reversed and nurses (including midwives here) are the primary care-givers (Kennell *et al.*, 1970). This serves to diminish her self-esteem, by persuading her that she is incompetent and, hence, superfluous in the care of her own child (Breen, 1978).

Larger NNUs usually comprise a Neonatal Intensive Care Unit (NNICU) and a Special Care Baby Unit (SCBU); an NNICU is able to provide more complex life-support systems and, thus, has higher staffing ratios (Wolke, 1987a). In this chapter I consider the baby at risk of dying in an NNU; as such a baby would obviously need more intensive care, my focus is more towards the NNICU. Although the neonatal period ends after twenty-eight days, many babies in the NNU are much older, but are still at risk of developing health problems which may cause their death. To avoid confusion, I consider here babies who are born alive, but who may die in this setting, rather than those who die at a strictly defined age. I use the term 'newborn' to indicate this less precise meaning.

In many ways, the grief which arises from the death of a newborn is similar to grief at other times; but, as there are certain unique aspects, my focus here is on those features of loss in the NNU which cause it to differ from other forms of loss. I look, first, at the ways in which grieving a newborn is unique; next, at the help which is available to the bereaved parents. Then I consider decision-making about continuing care in this area and, finally, I look at the setting in which this care is provided and the extent to which the environment affects caring.

Grieving a newborn

There are many accounts of the unique nature of grieving a newborn, but Benfield *et al.* (1978) describe authoritatively yet poignantly parents' feelings. In their NNICU, over 700 babies are admitted annually, of whom almost 16% do not survive. Their sample comprised 50 couples returning to discuss their baby's post-mortem results. Perhaps because the post-mortem was instrumental in recruitment, the sample is atypical, being all white and predominantly middle-class.

Table 9.1 Characteristics of babies dying in an NNU (Benfield *et al.*, 1978).

Characteristic	Mean	Range
Age of death	7.6 days	4.5 hours – 42 days
Birth weight	1.994 kg	0.790 kg – 4.080 kg

Despite the biased characteristics of the parents, the babies' data lead us to believe that the reactions of the parents need not be atypical. Each parent was asked to indicate their measure of grief in seven key areas:

- feeling sad
- loss of appetite
- sleeplessness
- being more irritable
- being preoccupied with the dead baby
- feeling guilty about the baby's death
- feeling angry

On the basis of the responses to these items, the researchers drew up a grief score for every parent. This score was used to compare the grief of mothers and fathers, and to compare the grief of those who were more involved and those who were less involved in treatment decision-making.

These researchers concluded that grieving a newborn is a highly individual experience and is unrelated to birth weight, age/gestation of the baby at death, degree of parental contact, previous perinatal loss or parental age. Benfield used parents' additional comments to draw up a list of concerns, all of which were raised very frequently.

Anger, directed at both the staff and God, pervaded the experience of a large majority of the parents. It carried with it a significant element of blame, some of which was self-blame, commonly known as *guilt*. Although these researchers do not detail the source of the parents' guilt, Nichols (1986) notes a particular tendency for the mother to analyse all her activities in order to blame those which caused her child's death (Klaus & Kennell, 1982b). An example would be the mother's self-care, which may have been criticised during pregnancy because of smoking or resting insufficiently, and thus aggravates her guilt (Rapoport, 1981). This guilt-analysis may constitute part of grieving, being comparable with the bargaining noted by Kubler-Ross (1970).

Disbelief or unreality was also raised (Benfield *et al.*, 1978), which may relate to the rarity of death of a newborn, or at least to the veto on mentioning it socially. Alternatively, disbelief may indicate that some degree of denial still persists, as in the quote from a mother: 'I keep waiting for the phone to ring, to wake up from my sleep and hear my baby crying'.

These researchers also describe the *'awkward moments'* encountered by the grieving couple. These include the usually innocuous questions such as 'What did you have?' from a casual acquaintance or another mother in the maternity unit. More serious are the incidents attributable to failures in the health care system, such as the respondent whose obstetrician inquired after her baby's health (Benfield *et al.*, 1978). My own experience is that these 'awkward moments' still occur; such as when I was recently admitting a new mother to the postnatal ward, knowing that her 25-week baby was dying in the NNU. Her obstetric notes had stayed with her baby, so I did not even know the sex of her baby, let alone the details of the birth. My problems were compounded by my inability to speak her language.

In Benfield's study, the feelings aroused by the *post-mortem* (PM) emerged when the parents reported their uncertainty of whether to attend to learn of the result. Rapoport (1981) discusses some of the reasons for parents' decisions about a PM, including some seeking as much information as possible in the hope of preventing a recurrence. Those who decline permission for a PM may have a religious reason, or may fear that their baby will be used for 'experimentation'. Alternatively, parents may want their family to 'view the body' to assist their grieving, or they may feel that their baby has gone through enough already, without what they see as this final insult.

Factors that may make grieving a newborn less difficult

Although I question whether any form of grief is easy, some writers suggest that certain features of death of a newborn make grieving less difficult. An example is the idea that neonatal death is not so 'thought-stopping' as stillbirth (Lewis & Bourne, 1989). In contrast to the research by Benfield *et al.* (1978), these writers suggest that longer survival correlates with less bewilderment and that the horror and feeling of 'defilement' associated with stillbirth is absent.

They go on to state that grieving is assisted by having been able to see and hold the live baby and by the legal requirement for certification of both birth and death of a baby who has lived independently; both of which serve to make the death of a newborn more like other deaths and to reduce the risk of failed mourning. This view is supported by the suggestion that the greater involvement, and investment, of staff in the care of a dying newborn increases the likelihood of the parents being well-supported (Littlewood, 1992).

The tendency to regard death of a newborn as less deserving of grieving than the death of an older person is founded on the societal assumption that the limited contact with the newborn requires or engenders less grief. This assumption ignores the affection which the mother develops towards the baby prenatally. Comparing the ease or difficulty of one form of grief with another is dangerous. Grief is fundamentally individual and there may be other 'baggage' facing the parents which, unknown to us, affects their grieving. We should beware of trivialising or underestimating the significance of any experience of grief. It is necessary to accept that, as has been said of pain, grief 'is what the person experiencing it says it is' (McCaffery, 1979).

The likelihood of the death of a newborn being trivialised was demonstrated by a research project which studied the events and personal interactions which either helped or hindered seven couples' grieving (Helmrath & Steinitz, 1978). As well as confirming the differences in grieving between the mothers and the fathers, these researchers illuminated the extreme isolation of these parents from friends and family. Like Benfield *et al.*, feelings of guilt were found to prevail. The bereaved parents were distressed by the assumption that the death of a baby was essentially different from the loss of an older child, as evidenced by friends' insensitive comments and unwillingness to mention the baby.

Helmrath and Steinitz (1978) attribute this unhelpful behaviour to the belief that the baby is replaceable. Others' lack of contact with the baby leads them to feel that grief is misplaced. These observations lead the authors to suggest that the bereaved parents should recognise their loss and grieve as *they* feel necessary.

Factors that may make grieving a newborn more difficult

As I have shown already, others' tendency to underestimate the significance of the death of a newborn in itself constitutes a barrier to grieving. There are a number of other factors which may further impede grieving.

The difficulty of the mother making contact with her ill baby is aggravated by the likelihood that she is being cared for in the maternity unit and her child is in the NNU which may be distant. This problem will be further compounded by her immobility if the birth was by caesarean section or she has an otherwise incapacitating problem.

Benfield *et al.* (1978) discuss the mother and baby being in different hospitals, suggesting geographical distance. Lack of communication, and perhaps trust, between the staff of different units also emerge in this paper: '. . . the referring hospital adversely influenced parent grieving', and, 'her obstetrician inquired about her baby's health . . . her baby had died three weeks earlier'. Such poor communication can in no way facilitate grieving and may have the reverse effect.

Nichols (1986) discusses the rationale for transferring an ill baby away from the mother soon after birth, without having given the mother an opportunity to get to know her child. This is less of a problem when the mother gives birth in a conurbation, where transport is easy, but it may carry considerable cost implications in more isolated areas.

Kennell and Klaus (1982) emphasise the need for mother and baby to be transferred together to a unit with the necessary NNU; this minimises family disruption. These authors show how neonatal mortality is reduced by *in utero* transfers, and then go on to describe their new regime for transporting the 'healthy premature' infant to be with the mother in the maternity unit. Although the healthiness of these babies excludes them from the group on which I am focusing, it is necessary to ask whether this more relaxed contact, being closely supervised with resuscitation equipment at hand, might be equally beneficial to less healthy babies and their mothers.

The geographical difficulties associated with the mother still remaining in the maternity unit become particularly acute should the baby die. The mother's non-involvement in arranging her baby's funeral while she is still in hospital may be a deliberate ploy to spare her pain (Nichols, 1986), in which family and undertakers collude for her presumed welfare. Benfield *et al.* (1978) stress that the mother's wishes about the funeral should not be ignored; they recommend postponing the funeral until the mother is fit to participate or holding a service in her hospital room.

Although it is unusual for a mother to be too unwell to attend the funeral, I have known mothers who have found this difficult. One mother who had a long-standing wound infection appreciated the importance of attending the service and was eventually supported by her family in making the journey. Another mother, a devout Muslim, was prevented by her 'unclean' status from attending, while making a difficult recovery from her caesarean section.

Partly based on her personal experience as a bereaved parent, Nichols (1986) attributes many of the grieving problems encountered by parents of dying newborns to discounted grief and negated death. She cites the non-involvement of the mother in the funeral and the equation of no contact with no grief as examples. She quotes some hurtful cliches which reflect the negation of newborn death, such as 'You weren't *really* a mother, why are you acting this way?' Such negation deprives the bereaved parent of social support and inhibits the progress of grief work.

The unexpectedness of premature birth and newborn death further serve to impede grieving. Nichols, a bereavement consultant in an NNICU, (1986), reports that because half of the deaths in the unit happened within 68 hours of birth, the parents find themselves in a shocked and confused state. So much so that they feel uncertain whether they are grieving the baby of their pre-natal fantasies, or a baby who has actually been born. They are unable to differentiate where their hopes and dreams ended and where reality began.

Parents' confused state leads them to be uncertain about whether to build on their attachment to their ill baby. They are anxious that, in the event of the baby dying, their investment of love and affection will take its toll in grief. Their indecisiveness aggravates their guilt at not feeling an overwhelming surge of love for their baby (Moore, 1981). Kennell and Klaus (1982) link the parents' uncertainty about forming a relationship with their baby to the need to prepare themselves first for the possible loss of their child, that is, the need for anticipatory grieving.

Anticipatory grieving

The benefits and hazards of anticipatory grieving have been debated since Lindemann first introduced the term (1944). If we view anticipatory grieving prospectively, we see the benefits to the bereaved in terms of the gentle modification of grief when death does come, allowing equilibrium to be regained more easily (Fulton & Gottesman, 1980). Alternatively, looking at it retrospectively, the damage to the relationship is all too easily apparent if the dying person does not succumb.

Fulton and Gottesman warn us not to confuse anticipatory grieving with forewarning of loss. Whereas forewarning is simply that, anticipatory grieving comprises a complex interplay of psychological, physical and social factors which serve to make it crucially different from post-mortem grief. The psychological differences comprise the intensification of certain aspects of grief and the alleviation of others; so the depth of guilt, despondency and anger vary hugely. Non-recognition of anticipatory grieving reduces social interactions and social support to the bereaved person, at both the personal as well as the institutional or ritual level.

Although McHaffie (1988) states that anticipatory grieving is the first psychological task to face the mother of an ill newborn, it may be that this process begins even earlier. I have been with mothers beginning to grieve before their baby is even born, when they threaten to go into labour at 24 or 26 weeks. The negative potential of anticipatory grieving is explained by Richards (1983) when he, like Fulton & Gottesman (1980), observes that the emotional reactions to the birth of an at-risk newborn, such as depression and mourning, may jeopardise the mother's relationship with her new baby.

Anticipatory grieving in the parents of ill newborns was established by Benfield *et al.* (1976) in their study of 101 couples whose babies had been admitted to an NNICU. A questionnaire measuring the parents' level of grieving was completed by each of the parents when their child was discharged. Despite the effects of time on the parents' memories, almost all reacted in a way comparable with those parents whose baby had died. The questionnaire responses showed feelings, attitudes and behaviours which reflected all-too-clearly the confusion and ambivalence associated with hovering between developing affection and anticipatory grieving.

The vacillation within the parent as they try to make sense of their fluctuating emotions can only be compounded by their reactions to the unpredictable changes in their baby's condition. The improvements and setbacks in their baby's progress may be compared with the roller-coaster effect which is a well-known feature of grieving (Aradine & Ferketich, 1990).

Preparing the parents

While for some parents the birth of an ill baby and the baby's admission to the NNU will be an earth-shattering catastrophe, for others it may be less unpredictable. The woman who has been regarded as 'high-risk' during her pregnancy and who, with her fetus, has been through intensive antenatal monitoring (Fogel, 1981) will have been prepared for a less than normal outcome. She may have been admitted to the antenatal ward on a long-term basis, or she may have undergone monitoring in a day assessment unit.

Either way, the opportunity should have been grasped to prepare her for the likely care of her baby in the NNU. The NNU staff are able to meet with parents to discuss anxieties and potential problems and to arrange a visit to the area of the NNU where their baby is likely to be cared for (Boxall & Whitby, 1983). The neonatal nurse is ideally suited to introduce the parents to both the physical environment and some of the staff who will be caring for their baby. Adopting an appropriately cautious or encouraging approach, the nurse explains the techniques and equipment which may be used; she may include the 'rogue's gallery', showing babies after they have gone home.

Parental involvement in care

When caring for parents with babies in the NNU we aim to provide a setting in which they are able to grieve their loss and form a close, loving relationship with their newborn (Lancaster, 1981). To help them to come to accept the reality of their situation, they may be gently encouraged to see, hold and care for their baby from its earliest moments. This involvement helps them, if and when it becomes necessary, to grieve for a specific baby, rather than for some vague entity which they never knew and are unable to recall or visualise (Moore, 1981).

Kennell and Klaus (1982) show us the importance of emphasising to the mother the positive aspects of her involvement with baby care. Whereas she may feel incompetent or even fearful of harming her baby, we should explain the benefits of her contact with her baby. Thus, welcoming the involvement of the mother in her baby's care is essential. We have to ensure that caring interventions which she is able to perform, such as feeding, should be certain to be successful. Thus, we help her to build up her self-confidence and self-esteem, to ensure an emotional environment in which the mother–child relationship can flourish.

Communication

Communication between staff and parents is crucial in this setting. We need to think about the information and support needs of the parents, their difficulty in accepting the 'bad news' and some practical aspects of facilitating communication.

Information-giving

Initially, we prepare the parents for the baby's appearance and the battery of surrounding equipment; later, we encourage the parents to share their concerns about their role and their baby's progress, while information-giving continues. The information given to the parents at their baby's admission may be supplemented by a booklet covering similar areas (Jacques *et al.*, 1983). To decide when we should be present with the family or absent, we have to balance the need to be supportive with the intimacy of the developing relationship.

Breaking the bad news

When we inform parents of the anticipated death of their newborn, we need to take account of our own feelings of disappointment and failure as well as the parents' grief. Waller *et al.* (1979) discuss the problems of the paediatrician who is faced with hostile denial in the parents of a dying child. While denial is a helpful coping mechanism when used on a temporary basis, persistent denial indicates that grief work is not progressing. An excessive degree of denial, as manifested by hostility and aggression, indicates that the unbearable pain of the reality persists.

After contemplating the possibility of not giving the bad news until the parents actually ask for it, these authors suggest guidelines to avoid this *impasse*. They recommend that information should be given with tact and sensitivity to its acceptance. Further information should only be given after checking the parents' understanding and acceptance of what they have been told already.

On the grounds that the degree of denial varies according to whether the staff member giving the news has a nursing or a medical background, consultation between the team of carers may provide insights into the parents' understanding. Denial may be a plea for greater support to help them to accept what they are being told.

Facilitating communication

Parents' anxieties relate to both the welfare of their baby and to their own functioning as parents. Self-doubt may inhibit parents from seeking information about or contact with their child, so it is essential that NNU staff should 'go the extra mile' in order to ensure that the parents do keep in touch. This may be by providing a free telephone line through which parents may obtain up-to-date information from NNU nursing staff about progress (Nichols, 1986; Benfield *et al.*, 1978). Similarly, personal family contact (McHaffie, 1992) may be encouraged by genuine 24 hour visiting, without anxiety-provoking delays before being allowed to enter the unit.

Changing practices in an NNU

Jacques *et al.* (1983) describe the procedures which they introduced in an NNU to facilitate the mother's feelings of closeness to her low birth weight (LBW) baby. Fundamental to these changes was a change of attitude among the caring staff towards acceptance and inclusion of the parents. The interventions included giving parents:

(1) an explanatory booklet outlining problems common to LBW babies
(2) a Polaroid photograph of their baby
(3) more encouragement to visit, hold and care for their baby
(4) two opportunities to discuss their baby's health with a paediatrician
(5) facilities to 'room in' with their baby before discharge
(6) intensive health visiting support.

Changing the care of the dying baby and the family

Many of these examples of family centred care may be applied to babies who are dying, as well as to healthier newborns. Harmon *et al.* (1984)

implemented more palliative concepts of hospice care to an NNICU, which resulted in, first, aggressive medical interventions being used more cautiously, second, more attention being given to a comfortable atmosphere in the unit and, third, a greater focus on the needs of the family, such as a family room for being with a dying or dead baby. The mothers on this programme found it helpful.

The need for interventions such as those used by Harmon *et al.* is made all too clear by the work of White *et al.* (1984) which studied the way in which death and parental grief is handled in an SCBU. Of 17 families approached, 12 agreed to be interviewed between 2 months and 13 months after their baby died. The researchers found that some of the parents were offered mementoes of their dead baby, such as a name-band, a cot card or a lock of hair. Five families accepted these items and three families regretted having no memento. Two families were forced to resort to secretly taking something belonging to their baby.

Ten of the families were satisfied with the way the loss had been handled, but White *et al.* found that two families felt that communication had been inadequate. The particularly poor communication after the death demonstrated, yet again, the difficulty which carers have in coping with death. This conclusion is supported by the observation that, despite their commitment to long-term family care, all the families' GPs preferred the NNU staff to undertake the bereavement counselling.

The lack of support for grieving parents became apparent in the 7 families who would have appreciated some form of mutual support, but who had no information about such help. Family support was good for 10 of the couples, which was just as well because one mother was not visited by any of the 'caring professions'. Others were visited by a range of personnel, including health visitors, midwives, GPs and priests.

Carers may seek to 'overprotect' the bereaved mother by hiding the extent of her baby's difficulties (Nichols, 1986). Whether it is actually the mother who is being protected is questionable, as the carers may be avoiding embarrassing displays of overt grief. Well-meaning family and friends may also 'overprotect' the mother by discouraging her from attending the funeral and putting her baby equipment out of sight.

Dissatisfaction with the traditional tendency to 'overprotect' the mothers helped to initiate the research project which increased parental involvement in NNUs and 'opened up' this topic (Kennell *et al.*, 1970). Twenty mothers who had had physical contact with their live newborns agreed to be involved after the babies survived between 1 hour and 12 days. The interviews focused on the birth experience and the baby's death, followed (for 13 mothers) by a questionnaire. A grief score was calculated for each mother and was correlated with her experience.

As well as showing that mothers encounter no ill-effects attributable to touching or holding their babies, this study indicated that hospital policies regarding these mothers' care needed attention. Contact with the mothers of healthy babies was unwelcome, and, although the grieving mothers could deal with other mothers' casual enquiries, the 'awkward moments' (Benfield *et al.*, 1978) due to staff ignorance were disturbing.

Optimism led the parents to interpret casual remarks from junior medical staff as predicting survival. This interpretation included some elements of magical thinking: 'If the baby survives for ... days, he will not die'. The parents were frequently tragically disappointed.

This study discounted earlier assumptions that mother-love suddenly develops when a mother sees or touches her newborn, by demonstrating affectional ties well in advance of seeing or having physical contact. Previous practices, such as hastily removing stillborn babies from their mothers' presence or discouraging mothers' access to their sick or dying babies, were shown to be unhelpful. By discussing its social dimensions, these researchers remind us that the death of a newborn is considerably more than a medical event.

Social and staff support

The social dimensions of care of newborns extend far beyond the nuclear family and the staff. This was demonstrated in a study of social support for the parents of babies in a NNICU (McHaffie, 1992) which focused on the role of grandparents. Four main components of social support are usually differentiated:

- emotional support
- esteem-building
- instrumental support
- information-giving.

Using questionnaires, McHaffie sought the views of parents and grandparents, as well as NNU staff. In this study she highlighted some of the 'mismatches' between staff expectations and grandparents' actual support. Their role is greatly and widely undervalued by staff, particularly by medical colleagues. If carers are to provide a milieu in which parents can relate to their newborn, they should encourage and utilise the parents' informal support system.

Although I look at staff support in the context of perinatal death in Chapter 9, I mention it briefly here because of specific relevant research and because of the implications of the unique NNU environment. Sherr (1989b) details the problems for NNU staff when a baby dies; as well as their professional feelings of failure, the staff grieve the death of a person with whom, over a period of hours, days or weeks, they have developed a caring relationship.

Coping mechanisms

Describing a staff support group, Bender and Swan-Parente (1983) focus on the problems faced by NNU staff, particularly how they cope with the psychological stress, pain and conflict engendered through care of newborns.

Denial and avoidance feature prominently among the short-term coping mechanisms, which these authors believe was reflected in their reluctance to meet to discuss their work-related stresses. Magical thinking and intuition were also identified, such as the 'unlucky incubator'. Staff also use projection and splitting, involving blaming others (including objects) for events for which they felt responsible. Examples which these authors mention and which I have already mentioned include blaming the obstetrician or the other hospital for less than optimal care.

Less experienced and junior staff identify with the parents in their feelings of inadequacy, incompetence and ignorance. Likewise, feelings of distress in the staff may be uncomfortably similar to those that they imagine are being felt by the baby. Feelings of rivalry, perhaps to be expected in an inexperienced and vulnerable mother whose baby is being nursed by super-competent staff, are also experienced by these staff. This reflects attachment which is an inevitable consequence of the long-term close contact of staff with a few ill newborns, which may be aggravated as primary nursing becomes more widespread.

A staff group

Her experience of establishing a staff group to help cope with these feelings is recounted by Bender (1981). Despite staff appearing enthusiastic for support, the group took 'many months' of perseverance to become established.

Organisational difficulties, such as staff rotation and shift working, tended to be blamed. Bender, however, believes that low morale and unacknowledged stress gave 'just talking' too low a priority. Rather than being supportive, the staff perceived the group as being yet another pressure beyond their control.

Bender reflects on her feelings of hopelessness, impotence, isolation and rejection at being unable to get the group established, and considers that these feelings may have much in common with those of NNU staff caring for dying newborns. In her evaluation of this group, Bender concludes the following:

(1) she managed to create a forum for staff to express conflicts and anxieties
(2) these meetings could focus on policy matters

(3) she identified and helped resolve conflicts such as bereavement and attachment
(4) appreciation of the babies' psychological and emotional needs increased, as exemplified by falling opposition to dummies being used as comforters.

Communication between parents

The feelings of isolation engendered in each parent with an ill newborn make it unsurprising that their relationship undergoes considerable strain. Their difficulty in sharing their feelings about their experience is compounded by this stress.

In their study of mothers grieving the death of a newborn, Kennell *et al.* (1970) found that mothers having difficulty mourning their loss reported being unable to talk to those close to them, such as their partners. Those mothers who had been able to share their feelings of loss were better able to work through their grief. It is necessary to question whether the difficulty originates in the relationship or in the experience of loss. That the relationship has difficulties is indicated by the observation that the mothers who were grieving less well had tried to broach the topic with their partners but 'had been ignored or cut off'.

These researchers' findings are confirmed by White *et al.* (1984) in their study of 12 families grieving the death of a newborn. They found that mothers whose grief was progressing less well were in less supportive relationships. Unfortunately, research focusing on the negative aspects of the parents' relationship is unable to show us whether the relationship was weak before the birth or whether the baby's admission has affected it.

Like Kennell *et al.*, Helmrath and Steinitz (1978) identified benefits in better communication between parents. They also found that bereaved parents who were able to share their feelings experienced an increase in their mutual trust which they felt was essential to the resolution of their grief. The couples also thought that the quality of their relationship had improved and perceived their loss as having been an opportunity for growth.

Decision-making: initiating and continuing treatment

In providing care for the family and their newborn, carers aim to sustain life and alleviate suffering. Ordinarily these aims are mutually compatible, but sometimes there may be conflict. An example is the LBW baby whose healthy development is jeopardised by a variety of pathological and other insults. Questions arise about whether and for how long treatment should be continued, about who should take the decision and how it should be made. In some countries these decisions have been assumed by the legislature (Caplan *et al.*, 1992), but in the UK the 'situation is not at all clear' (Richards, 1987). Although euthanasia *may* be relevant, I am focusing on treatment-related decisions because, although the outcome may be similar, the decisions, intentionality and procedures are not.

Initiation of treatment

The seriously ill newborn in the NNU may have been resuscitated in the birthing room or the baby may have begun breathing spontaneously. Either way, the baby's independent existence has become established. Any other course of action would be inappropriate, because the labour ward is not the ideal place to make unexpected life-and-death decisions, due to the limited time to either confer with the parents or make a complete assessment of the baby's condition.

Unfortunately, when the baby is transferred to the NNU a sequence of interventions has begun which assumes a momentum of its own. In their study of aggressive neonatal care, Guillemin and Holmstrom (1986) describe this form of incrementalism as the 'all or none' law. I question whether this policy constitutes humane care (Penticuff, 1992).

Resource implications

Bound up with continuation of treatment are issues relating to resource allocation. Without disregarding the financial costs of caring for a sick newborn for possibly months, one should also consider what is foregone. By providing NNU care for a baby born at 24 weeks, we deny care to three babies born at 32 weeks. It is necessary to ask whether decision-making on a 'first come, first served' basis is ideal.

Decision-making – by whom?

Who makes the decision about continuing treatment may affect the outcome of that decision. Medical staff focus on the immediate situation and the problems as they present in the NNU, whereas their nursing colleagues are better able to adopt a 'holistic view' (Guillemin & Holmstrom, 1986). Thus, nurses think of the baby becoming a child and a person in a social context and the family resources to care for someone growing up with potentially severe disabilities. This point is not unrelated to the earlier 'incrementalist' argument, because staff who have worked hard to sustain a newborn may have difficulty in abandoning all the effort and emotion that they have invested.

The involvement of parents in treatment decision-making is debated on the grounds that such responsibility is hard to bear (Borg & Lasker, 1982). The grieving of 19 parents who had shared the decision to limit care was compared with the grieving of 21 parents whose babies had received total care (Benfield *et al.*, 1978). The mothers of the limited care babies demonstrated significantly less anger, irritability and 'wanting to be left alone'. The fathers in the limited care group encountered less sleeplessness, irritability, depression, crying and loss of appetite. Thus, while some parents may avoid such involvement, well-informed parents are able to contribute to taxing decisions about treatment and go on to adjust healthily to their loss.

Having contemplated the limitations of legislation in offering a suitable framework for these difficult decisions (Caplan *et al.*, 1992), we must consider using multidisciplinary decision-making committees. Richards (1987) recounts the previous lack of success of such committees, but concludes that we should 'persist and try different structures'.

Davis (1983) reviews extreme approaches to decision-making, with the backing of law at one end and total parental discretion at the other. He suggests a 'middle ground' or consensus in which the rights, needs, responsibilities and feelings of *all* concerned are taken into account in each individual situation. Openness in this form of decision-making would maintain the confidence of all who are involved and, particularly important, the public.

Care after the decision to discontinue treatment

After emphasising the need to focus on 'the best interests of the infant' and the benefits of parental involvement in caring for a dying baby after deciding to discontinue life-sustaining treatment, de Leeuw (1989) discusses the benefits for the baby of using analgesic or sedative drugs. He acknowledges the likelihood of death being hastened, but argues the humanity of this medication. The parents are involved whenever possible in a private setting, together with other chosen family members. Supporting the parents through the baby's dying and laying-out is essential, in the hope that they appreciate the naturalness of death as an essential feature of life.

The setting in which care happens

Up to this point in this chapter we have been thinking about the processes and events which take place in the NNU. These include beginning relationships, ending others, loving, supporting as well as making hard decisions. I would like now to focus on the environment in which all these happen and which inevitably affects them, starting with the intimate environment in which the baby is treated and moving on to the more general environment in which parents and staff interact.

Touch and handling

The benefits of tactile stimulation to a newborn are well-established (Solkoff *et al.*, 1969). Likewise, parental care involves handling as part of affectionate social interaction (Murdoch & Darlow, 1984). However, emphasising the importance of rest for LBW and sick newborns, Wolke (1987a) reminds us of the iatrogenic effects of excessive manipulation during monitoring and other procedures, including hypoxaemia, bradycardia, apnoea and behavioural distress.

In their intensive observational study of 11 extremely LBW babies, Werner and Conway (1990) recorded contacts during 20 hours of care. The mean gestational age of the babies observed was 26.3 weeks, their mean chronological age was 4.6 hours and their mean birthweight 0.891 kg. These researchers categorised contacts according to whether they were direct, therapeutic or incidental.

Disconcertingly, these researchers found that the most vulnerable babies were exposed to the greatest number of indirect contacts; to the extent that those with a 'minimal touch' instruction were disturbed approximately twice as often as those without. Werner and Conway challenge nurses to plan and coordinate their care to minimise disruption and maximise comfort activities.

The purely physical benefits of the LBW newborn's immediate environment are considered by Turrill (1992). She discusses the effects of being born prematurely on the infant's perception of and relationship with the immediate environment. This baby is deprived of pressure from the uterine walls which the fetus ordinarily experiences due, first, to the walls' increasing contractility and, second, to the relative reduction in amniotic fluid. The effect of extrauterine gravity has more marked effects on the relatively hypotonic newborn musculature. Thus, normal sensorimotor development is impeded, unless deliberate precautions are taken to imitate the natural phenomena by correct positioning and other interventions.

The possibility of using a pile decubitus pad to imitate normally-occurring intrauterine tactile stimulation was investigated by Nelson *et al.* (1986). The pad was intended to substitute for the positive touch techniques which have been shown to facilitate physiological and emotional development. The authors had to conclude that this form of pad alone was insufficient to imitate the human contact of which LBW newborns are deprived. This intervention, like the much-publicised Kangaroo care, needs more research before being recommended for the care of small, sick or dying babies.

The wider environment

Although they avoid the word, Werner and Conway (1990) demonstrated the stressors which are inadvertently applied by carers in the

NNU and which may affect the condition of a dying baby or the care that baby receives. The stressors caused physical as well as psychological stress through interrupting sleep and rest.

Using complex monitoring equipment, Horsley (1990) studied three aspects of the physical environment in the NNU: noise, light and handling. She found that although the background noise levels inside incubators were within the recommended limit (60 decibels), impact noises such as closing port-holes increased this to almost 80 decibels. She was unable to measure the effect of continuous pop music on the newborn. Horsley showed that light levels experienced by newborns equated with levels found to cause retinal damage in experimental animals and occasionally 'far exceeded' operating theatre levels. Her findings relating to handling concur with those mentioned already.

Developmental factors

In his paper on 'environmental neonatology', Wolke (1987b) discusses the effects of negative stimuli, such as 'noise pollution', on newborn development. He emphasises not just the health risks which may result, but also the effect of the incubator in diffusing sound, thus preventing the newborn from associating, for example, a face with a particular voice. The newborn is thus deprived of learning opportunities. While regretting our limited knowledge of the effects of *excessive* light, Wolke relates the lack of a diurnal pattern of light in the NNU to later sleeping problems.

Having recognised the largely negative stimuli to which the newborn is exposed, Wolke (1987b) highlights the inappropriateness of these stimuli to learning and psychological development. He shows that, perhaps because of a decreased staffing ratio, nurses 'do not change' their approach to the older newborn to take account of developing abilities. He blames this inflexibility for the interactional problems encountered later. On the basis of these observations he recommends (1987a) that we should:

(1) observe each newborn more closely for sociable behaviour as well as signs of disorganisation
(2) individualise care
(3) 'grow up with the patient'.

Changing attitudes

Concerns about the harmful effects of NNUs on newborn development underlie research by Becker *et al.* (1991). They discuss the stressful NNU environment and, like Wolke (1987a, b), its potential for impeding learning. These researchers also advocate an individualised developmental approach to care.

To evaluate this approach they designed an experimental study comparing growth and behavioural organisation outcome measures in two groups of very LBW babies. The first group of 21 newborns acted as controls. The second, experimental group of 24 were cared for by nurses who had been educated both didactically and individually to reduce environmental stressors by:

- limiting light and sound
- providing comfort during interventions, such as by using a dummy
- promoting sleep/wake organisation by planning/clustering interventions
- giving postural support through 'nesters'
- encouraging non-nutritive sucking while tube-feeding.

Newborns in the experimental group had fewer respiratory and feeding problems, lower morbidity, shorter admission times and better behavioural organisation. These outcomes indicate that education of nurses to take account of environmental and psychological factors does affect newborn well-being.

The NNU environment

Considerable research has focused on the setting in which care of the LBW and ill newborn is provided. The hazards that have been identified and the outcomes that have been measured relate to the well-being of the newborn. The NNU as a working environment has been given little attention.

Exceptionally, a comparative study was undertaken of staff perceptions of two ward environments: an NNU and an orthopaedic ward (Spinks & Michaelson, 1989). The NNU staff showed marked dissatisfaction with their working conditions. This applied to many organisational factors such as lack of autonomy and poor interpersonal relationships; but they felt strongly that the organisational difficulties were aggravated by physical discomfort, engendering unacceptably high stress levels, high temperature being an example of physical discomfort.

Summary

'All human life is there' in the NNU, and a lot more besides. I have shown that the NNU is for living, loving and dying, for finding and losing, for helping to live and allowing to die. These activities continue to happen regardless of the environment. I have shown the efforts which are being made to improve the environment for the babies beginning and perhaps ending their lives there and what is being done to improve the experience of their parents and family. The staff are crucial in helping parents to adjust to the possible loss of their hopes and expectations through the loss of their baby. Whether we provide the healthiest environment in which the staff are able to facilitate all these activities is unclear.

Chapter 9
Staff Reactions and Support

Observing reactions to the loss of a baby, a psychiatrist describes how staff are 'flung apart' by such a loss (Bourne, 1979). In this chapter I look at how members of staff are or are not able to cope with the experience of being 'flung apart' and the solutions which have been suggested to help them.

Mallinson (1989) shows the relevance of Bourne's observation to midwives in her account of how, in hospital, a dead baby is likely to have been quickly removed from the presence of the mother. The rationale for this hasty removal was founded on the then widespread mis-understanding of the twin processes of bonding and grieving, leading to a misplaced desire to protect the mother from further anguish.

This misunderstanding is implicit in the subsequent comments by Bourne in which, focusing on our medical colleagues, he reports the lack of research and literature relating to perinatal death. His own earlier research had identified the difficulty that some medical prac-titioners face when a baby dies; as evidenced by the inability of general practitioners to recall even basic factual information, such as the names of families in which a baby has died (Bourne, 1968).

The reason for the significance of the reaction of the member of staff is spelt out by Osterweis et al. (1984). They suggest that health care personnel cannot be expected to provide optimal care and support for the dying and the grieving unless allowance is made for both their personal or family tensions and their occupational, especially grief-related, problems. The need for us as carers to be emotionally secure has also been raised in more general situations. For example, Cole (1993) suggests that 'in order to have healthy patients you need to have healthy staff'. Thus, it may be that emotional health is a fundamental requirement for those who provide care in stressful situations.

The reasons why members of staff may experience difficulty in coping with a perinatal death are threefold. First, on a personal level, we find the death of a baby shocking because it is untimely, that is, contrary to the normal cycle of birth, life and death (Worden, 1992). Although we know that we are likely to grieve the death of our parents, parents do not expect to have to mourn the death of their children. Perhaps because of this untimeliness, the loss of a baby raises many deeply-felt, long-hidden and perhaps unrecognised emotions, which may be associated with our memories and anticipations of past and future intimate losses (Kowalski, 1987).

Second, on a professional level, the loss of a baby represents a failure in our abilities as carers to perform that function which our chosen occupation requires of us – assisting with the birth of healthy babies. The fact that perinatal death has been entitled 'the ultimate defeat' (Queenan, 1978) indicates the difficulty which some may encounter in assisting with the care of a baby who is not alive and healthy.

This perception of failure in care gives rise to negative feelings among professionals, which have been identified by Stack (1982) in terms of helplessness, defeat, guilt, resentment and failure. The prospect of the death of a baby and the negative feelings arising from it may result in the desire to avoid that death at any cost (Peppers & Knapp, 1982). This avoidance develops into a confrontation in which carers may have to face the 'ultimate defeat' mentioned already.

Third, in terms of our learning, we tend to practise and become more skilled in doing those things in which we have been trained or in which we have experience; the corollary of this is that if we have not been trained or have not become experienced in handling a particular situation, we will not only not learn about it, but we may seek to avoid situations exposing our deficiency and the anxiety it engenders.

Buckman (1993) applies this rationale to the care of the dying adult, but it is not difficult to find similarities with our care for a grieving mother. He concludes that areas that are 'out of bounds' early in our careers may remain so throughout our working lives. We may surmise that this sequence may continue indefinitely on a cyclical basis if the insecurity and anxiety which these 'no go' areas engender is passed on to future generations of carers for whose education we are responsible.

It is clear that for any or all of these reasons, we may find ourselves fundamentally, and possibly disconcertingly deeply, affected when a baby is lost. Whether we are able to recognise in ourselves the extent to which we are personally affected by such a loss is less clear. The need to identify and acknowledge the personal implications of a death is fundamental to being able to care effectively for those who are dying and grieving (Osterweis *et al.*, 1984). These authors go on to explain the likely effects if this need is not adequately met, showing how 'stress can escalate quickly'.

Stress

The stress experienced by nurses caring for dying adults in acute hospital wards was identified by Hockley (1989). She describes how all the nurses found contact with the dying person and their relatives stressful. However, 60% of her sample identified the rewarding nature of this form of care.

The extent to which caring for a grieving mother is stressful for us as carers emerged during my research (Mander, 1992d). In the course of her interview, Kay explained that for midwives the stress of grief is likely to be superimposed on the usually tolerable stress level associated with conscientious practice:

> *Kay*   It's a difficult situation . . . It's a situation of grief; anybody who's trained as a nurse will tell you that working with people who are dying is a very stressful occupation. Midwifery per se – delivering healthy babies – is stressful 'cos there's always the worry of 'I hope everything's all right'.

The way in which Kay talked about stress reflects our current general usage of this word. We tend to perceive stress as a uniformly negative phenomenon arising from a range of unpleasant experiences to which we are subjected (Bailey & Clarke, 1991).

This perception of the invariably negative nature of stress was called into question by the work of Selye (1956), when he looked at stress in physiological terms and concluded that it is a universal adaptive response. He named this response the general adaptation syndrome, or 'GAS'. Although many of our ideas about stress have moved on since Selye undertook his work, we should give him credit for his emphasis on the likelihood of stress being a response to a range of possibly threatening, challenging or enjoyable stimuli (Selye, 1980).

Selye's account of the nature of stress neglected the significance of individual factors, such as emotional and physiological characteristics, in the interpretation of stress. The interactionist explanation of stress is now more generally accepted (Lazarus, 1976), which regards stress as a product which arises out of the interaction between relevant features of the environment and the person who is perceiving the situation.

The interactionist view recognises that different people interpret the same situation as threatening, challenging or enjoyable to differing extents. The interpretation of the same person may also differ, possibly over time, associated with learning about a situation or possibly due to other factors which make the person more or less vulnerable.

A crucial feature of the interactionist view of stress is the significance of the *person's* interpretation of the situation in which they find themselves. We need to be wary of belittling another person's perception of the stress they experience – as with certain other phenomena we should accept that it is what the person experiencing it says it is. Holland (1987) shows the practical benefits of this approach by describing how, in a research setting, incorporating the interactionist view of stress resulted in group members assuming a more supportive and helpful approach to those with whom they worked. Among other benefits, this approach helped the participants to understand their shared feelings of stress.

The stress which is experienced by those staff involved in the loss of a baby is a topic which has been widely neglected. The reaction of the nurse caring for an adult who is dying has been studied in North America and the reactions of student nurses have been studied in the UK (Bailey & Clarke, 1991). These authors suggest that the response of the nurse to the death of a patient is variable and includes positive as well as negative elements. The positive aspects include feelings of the nurse having done her best for the patient or having helped the relatives in the most appropriate way. The less positive aspects may include any of the emotions which we face when a person dies.

Bailey and Clarke (1991) discuss the relative merits of the nurse being older and/or more experienced in helping her to perceive death and dying as less negatively stressful. In her research, Hockley (1989) found that experience made little difference to the degree of anxiety the nurse feels when caring for a dying adult, but the focus of that anxiety does differ. Those nurses with less experience tend to be more concerned about controlling their emotions, whereas more experienced nurses worry about their responsibility to the patient and their relatives.

Judging the value of age and experience in coping with perinatal death is even harder. This is because it is complicated by, first, the way in which we as carers in the maternity area identify strongly with those we care for and, second, the not insignificant input of personal experience to our care (Mander, 1992b).

Factors contributing to stress

Certain features, the midwives in my study told me, exacerbated their perception of stress associated with the loss of a baby. These features increased their vulnerability and, as suggested by Osterweis *et al.*, may have compromised the care they were able to provide for the grieving mother.

Difficulty dealing with grieving parents

The midwives described the challenge which caring for a grieving mother presents; this relates to the threefold difficulties of untimeliness, professional failure and unpreparedness mentioned already. Although learning about a situation may lower the stress which it engenders, Hattie, a midwife with many years' experience, told me how caring for grieving mothers did not become easier for her:

Hattie No matter how many of these mothers you deal with, it's always a very difficult situation. It's not easy having to cope with your own emotions and to care for the mother as well.

As mentioned by Osterweis *et al.* (1984), it may be difficult for us as carers to recognise our own emotions, which is clearly a prerequisite if we are to provide effective care through good communication:

Betty   It's hard for them and it's hard for us to talk about the death, so we have to work hard to build up a relationship in which they can express their feelings.

Occasionally the non-verbal messages given by the midwife warned me that her difficulties with even discussing the grieving mother were too sensitive for me to probe any further:

Florrie   I think it is a personal thing with me. It is not something I would like to have to deal with. I would find it quite difficult.

A perceptive comment by Queeny about the difficulty of staff in caring for the grieving mother, was accompanied by a facial expression which suggested that she was aware that what she was saying might not be generally acceptable:

Queeny   I can't help feeling that sometimes the staff have difficulty caring for this woman and this may be part of the reason for her getting home so soon.

Queeny's comment endorses my earlier suggestion that our difficulties in caring for the grieving mother may be associated with our sense of failure and may lead to avoidance of further potentially painful encounters. The possibility that we use discharge as a coping mechanism is also suggested by Kellner and Lake (1986), although the midwives I interviewed, with only the exception of Queeny, believed that it is the mother who decides when she returns home. If my informants had any thoughts about the relative merits of the mother grieving at home or in hospital, they considered that home was the more appropriate place, as family support would be more helpful.

The problems that we encounter when communicating with dying people and their relatives are well-known (Lugton, 1989). Fanny spelled out the feelings shared by the midwives I interviewed:

Fanny   I find a lot of times it's very difficult to know what to say to them. Obviously, you don't want to upset them any more than they already are. Sometimes it's difficult to know whether they want to talk about it or whether they don't want to talk about it. I think that's very difficult. But they need to talk.

Midwives told me how, normally, they use the prospect of the mother having a healthy baby to encourage her during her labour. Being unable to use this form of encouragement was sadly missed and caused the midwife to experience difficulty which would aggravate any pre-existing stress:

Irene   Usually when I'm caring for women in labour, I take a very positive approach and tell them that their contractions are bringing them nearer to the birth of the baby . . . you can't say this and so it is difficult to encourage her, so it has to be more a case of 'one pain at a time'.

Josie   . . . it is sometimes very difficult. You've got to keep reminding yourself not to keep saying 'You're going to have a happy little bundle at the end of it' and 'You'll look forward to looking after it'. Things like that, you've got to watch . . .

Having to 'watch' what she said in this way acted as a further source of stress with which the midwife had to cope.

Those midwives who worked primarily in the community encountered difficulties which might have been solved relatively simply, such as the daily postnatal check which is usually undertaken in the mother's home. Grieving parents were said to have assumed that the midwife is there to examine the baby; this apparent error in care may cause further unhappiness if the parents are not warned that the midwife will be coming to visit the mother.

Although some of the difficulties we encounter when caring for grieving parents are fundamentally profound, others are merely organisational matters which are easily solved or, preferably, prevented.

Lack of a happy outcome

Some of the staff who work in the maternity area are first attracted to it because they expect it to be a 'happy' area in which to work. Medical writers, such as Bourne (1979), are keenly aware of the relative rarity of perinatal death and that this may be seen as a benefit; he believes that the attraction of obstetrics lies in its healthy orientation and the possibility of 'some legitimate retreat from death and disease'. He goes on to spell out the unsuitability of this mental stance for the albeit rare perinatal deaths, the unhealthy consequences and the potential for psychiatrists to contribute more constructively.

Likewise, Peppers and Knapp (1982) describe the particular difficulty that physicians may have in dealing with death, requiring that it be avoided at all costs, going on to state that, for obstetricians and paediatricians, the acceptance of perinatal death may be especially fraught. This difficulty may be explained by the unrealistically high standards which medical staff may set themselves in their fight against perinatal deaths, resulting in the painful personal costs which have to be paid by the staff member (Klaus & Kennell, 1982b).

In their account of the education of health professionals about coping with death, Osterweis *et al.* (1984) regret the paucity of time spent in 'the training of physicians' on 'the personal reactions ... to illness, death and bereavement' and commend the way in which, in nursing courses, these are essential aspects of care.

The comments of Josie and Irene (above) indicate the way in which midwives perceive the need to behave in a different, perhaps less relaxed, way if the mother will be grieving not having her baby with her. The regret for the absence of the usual happy ending is apparent in a further comment by Josie:

Josie   Whereas with the lady who had an intrauterine death ... you haven't got a happy outcome at the end of it. It is a totally different situation you've actually got to cope with.

Unpreparedness to care for a mother who is grieving the loss of a baby may cause difficulties, especially for those who come into maternity care anticipating that it will be invariably enjoyable.

Mother's anger

An aspect of the grief reaction which exemplifies the contrast with the usual happy outcome and which carers find particularly hard to cope with is anger. Although her anger is largely unfocused, those who are with the mother on a 24 hour basis will inevitably be on the receiving end of these powerful emotions:

Nancy   Some people are really angry at first especially with hospital staff, they feel that maybe the hospital was at fault or whatever. Then some people just feel angry. I think that's part of the grieving process. I think you've just got to wait till the anger subsides and accept it.
Author   D'you find that a bit hard to take?
Nancy   I suppose that it is difficult but you've got to realise that it's just part and parcel of the whole process and not hold it against anyone for feeling that.

As well as the possibility of perceiving her anger as a personal insult, we have to consider its effect on our ability to care for the mother. Ruby indicates that it may act as a barrier to communication and, hence, caring:

Ruby   The staff may resent that so much of the anger is directed towards them. They have to get over that barrier initially.

While recognising the difficulty, Ginnie, indicates a mind set which helps her to work through the mother's superficial confrontational stance:

Ginnie Well, I don't think you would be human if you didn't [find the antag-
onism hard to take]. But you've got to remember that it is not directed
personally at you . . . y'know. I mean obviously this woman has had a very
traumatic experience, so I don't really find it hard to take. As I say you've
got to get to know the woman, it's very important.

Getting to know the woman, in spite of the antagonistic facade which
she presents, imposes heavy demands on the resources of those caring
for her. It is necessary now to consider the nature and adequacy of those
resources.

Limited resources

The care which we provide for the grieving mother is constrained in a
number of ways. The resources which we have at our disposal are finite,
unlike the demands which often appear infinite. In considering the
limitations on what we are able to offer the grieving mother, I focus,
first, on the personal factors which are integral to us as carers and,
second, on the organisational or more external facilities.

Personal factors

The midwives I interviewed were aware of their own shortcomings and
were far from complacent about their care:

Kay You just don't know what to tell a mother that's losing her baby or giving
birth to a baby that well may not live.

The midwives told me that part of their concern related to their limited
knowledge, which they attributed to inexperience due to the in-
frequency with which they encountered perinatal loss:

Trudy There is a great danger that the parents may be given incorrect
information about some aspect, particularly of the procedures involved.
This is probably because it is such an infrequent experience for each midwife and so she may not have very much knowledge about it.

Although our minds may inevitably turn first to the problems faced by
staff in the labour ward, those who work with mothers postnatally face
similar difficulties:

Nellie I can't say that I was particularly well prepared to cope. . . . I'd never
actually met a mother who'd lost her baby before. . . . I came on and was
told there was a mother who'd had a stillbirth and I remember the first time I
went in to see her and I thought I've got to see to this woman and I've got
nothing to say to this woman, there is nothing I can say to this woman to
help her. How do I cope with her and support her?

Wendy spelt out the feelings of inadequacy to which Nellie was referring:

Wendy   We're just not sure what to say in a situation such as that and we are frightened to put our foot in it and we're frightened of the reaction of the mum, [the midwife's] emotions are so fraught at these times, nervous, in case we say the wrong thing or do the wrong thing.

The midwives told me of how they thought that these feelings of inadequacy might be remedied:

Effie   I think at that time, having looked after somebody like that . . . and your own feelings of inadequacy at that time, you felt you wanted to go and read just to see if there was anything – what other views there were and what you should do in that situation.

Florrie   The other thing I would say is that we as midwives should have some special counselling or it should be necessary for all of us to attend some type of course, seminar or whatever so we are better equipped to deal with it. Because until I came to this [labour] ward about three months ago I had never come across these women.

Their lack of experience in caring for a grieving mother may be partly due to the practice in some units of only particular staff being involved. Clearly the expertise of the bereavement counsellor is helpful to the grieving mother, but other staff find their own anxieties and feelings of inadequacy are aggravated:

Queeny   I find, and I'm sure a lot of other midwives do, difficulty in treating this lady. This is because it's the [midwife manager] who counsels her and so the midwives don't get much opportunity to talk to her.

Organisational factors
In her research, Hockley (1989) found that nurses caring for adults who were dying experienced stress when they were unable, due to lack of time, to provide the care which they knew to be necessary. In the same way, the need to be able to spend time being available to the grieving mother caused many midwives to be acutely conscious of the pressures on their working time:

Deidre   In the . . . wards I think it is a bit more difficult because you have people coming up after having a stillbirth and often you have several patients to look after or you are in charge and you don't have a lot of time to spend with them, or not enough time.

This in turn made them realise the deficiencies in their care:

Nellie   We try our best to give them as much time to talk to us as possible. But I feel that really that isn't as good as we should be doing. We should be able to say 'I'm going to be here for an hour so let's sit down and talk about it'. What is really needed is more time to allow us to talk to these mothers and provide reassurance about the things that worry them. How we achieve this is not quite so easy; perhaps we need more staff, or it may be that we could do with less patients.

The difficulties the midwives faced in prioritising their work became overwhelmingly clear. Problems of resources were also recognised outside both the midwife's province and the health service:

Ginnie   I sometimes feel like banging my head off the wall. I can't give them enough support. My anger is with myself and with others, such as the social work departments – they don't have enough resources to care as much as these mothers need. Some of them are quite comfortably off while others have got nothing. I often feel frustrated that I am unable to do more for them. All these cutbacks mean that the mothers aren't getting so many milk tokens and because the milk firms have stopped giving out samples we can't even help them out with those any more.

The frustration clearly articulated by Ginnie was apparent in Kay's comments about the organisational resources available to support her:

Kay   It's very stressful and I think senior midwives, they often push someone in who they think can cope with the situation and leave them to it, without really realising that that midwife needs support as well. It's not easy. It's stressful. We're not talking about a normal day's work – it's not a normal day's work – this happens maybe once every six months to every midwife if they're very unfortunate, maybe less often. So I think they need support. I think very often you're just left to get on with it – just by sheer workload, y'know, of a unit. And I think senior midwives have got to realise that that person has got to get some TLC [tender loving care] as well.

Kay recognises that managers should make allowance for our need for 'tender loving care' in the same way that Niven (1992) draws our attention to the multiplicity of demands on health care professionals. She compares the stress experienced by a new mother in caring for and caring about her new baby with the stress that we may encounter when responding to the needs of the mothers in our care, as well as the demands of our lives outside our work. Although these non-work activities may be stressful in a negative sense, they may also provide us with an opportunity to 'recharge our batteries' and help us to get our work into perspective. This brings us to consider how we, as members of staff, are helped to cope with the stress of this aspect of our work.

Factors helping to alleviate stress

So far in this chapter I have shown that the difficulties that we encounter when a mother is grieving are due to the way in which factors within ourselves interact with factors in the environment. These difficulties were described by the midwives in my recent study in terms of 'stress' which they, like many others, perceived entirely negatively.

Stress may manifest itself in the early stages in the form of sickness absence or absenteeism, accidents or errors and in the later stages in what has become known as 'burnout' (Holland, 1987). We may regard sickness absence as coping strategy, which probably equates in terms of helpfulness with those listed by Lazarus (1976) including denial, escape, displacement and intellectualisation.

In this section we will be thinking about the more constructive and supportive methods which are used and have been suggested for adjusting to stress generally and to the stress of caring for a grieving mother in particular.

Our difficulty in receiving support from and giving support to our colleagues has been frequently observed (Chevenert, 1978; Crawley, 1983; Hillier, 1981; Hingley, 1984). Bond (1986) suggests that our own expectations and those of people near to us may prevent us from admitting our need for support. Additionally, an element of reaction formation may be present, through which we act 'in the opposite direction to an impulse or desire which is being repressed' (Drever, 1964). We may find either or both of these mechanisms in action to conceal our vulnerability.

The largely adverse press which peer support has received in the nursing culture has been summarised by Sutherland as 'a pejorative term which is applied only to people who are considered weak' (Cole, 1993). This observation appears to be supported by the experience of Annie:

Annie   There can be situations where the support [from my colleagues] would be lacking. I think that it is isolated, I don't think it is a general rule ... isolated incidences where support maybe wasn't there. I would say that all (this sounds terrible) – all the different kind of paperwork and everything, I would say you have a lot of help with that, but emotionally I wouldn't say that I have had particularly any help in that kind of way.

In spite of all these adverse observations, we can all call to mind occasions when we have found timely and effective support among our colleagues.

Peer support

Bond (1986) applies the concept of peer support to 'people who feel equal in status to one another' and goes on to relate this to similar levels in the nursing hierarchy. Although peers are the group that we would approach first when seeking support, it may be more appropriate to focus on the shared nature of the experience, rather than on the shared background of those experiencing it.

In keeping with this definition, I am considering peer support here in terms of the informal, *ad hoc*, or impromptu support which is uniquely relevant to the situation and the moment (Kowalski, 1987). It is the kind of help which is only needed, acceptable and appropriate for a fleeting moment and when that moment is past, similar offers of help seem clumsy, intrusive and embarrassing.

This kind of spontaneous spur-of-the-moment mutual support would include the widely-used 'waste paper basket' technique which involves little more than a good grumble. Tschudin (1982) states that this activity, like 'letting off steam' with which it has much in common, requires only a safe environment. 'Safety' in this context refers to the trustworthiness of the confidante.

An admirable example of this kind of on-the-spot support is provided by a general practitioner who found himself amid the Hillsborough disaster (Heller, 1993). After recognising the limitations of his own abilities in a situation of such overwhelming trauma, this GP was eventually able to identify many of his friends and colleagues feeling similarly inadequate. In spite of what we know about the macho attitudes of our medical colleagues, one of them, through this shared experience of inadequacy, was able to give him a totally unexpected yet very welcome hug, in recognition of what they had both been through on that day.

Kohner (1985) emphasises that a midwife who has just been involved with a grieving mother needs support, but that it must be support which is appropriate to the person who is seeking it. Whereas for Heller this 'support' took the form of physical contact, for others it may take the form of physical and psychological space in which to recover.

Although the literature tends to refer to the significance of one-to-one support, the midwives I interviewed seemed to consider themselves in terms of an informal group which was well able to support its members:

Ottily We all help and support each other when these things happen.
Hattie Midwives tend to help and support each other. Those who have been around for a longer time are better able to support the others and to share their feelings. This is done on quite an informal basis. There was one young midwife that I was able to help, she was in quite a state because she was qualified and during her training she had never seen a dead baby.
Irene My midwifery colleagues have always been supportive. The senior midwives were all right. They showed no sign of disapproving of you crying.

Although giving them only faint praise, Irene's comment leads us to consider the managers' role.

Managers' support

I have already alluded to the role of the manager in supporting those caring for a grieving mother in terms of expectations of staff being able to cope and also in the provision of adequate human resources; adequacy refers to the appropriate number of staff with the relevant skills. The need for the manager at the level of the ward or other clinical area to be aware of any emotional vulnerability in any of their staff is discussed in Chapter 10.

Lugton (1989) is one of the few writers who credits managers with any role in grieving situations. She recognises that one of these functions is for senior staff to serve as role models, possibly by encouraging other staff to accompany them when they are speaking with people who are dying or grieving. Lugton also highlights the role of managers in creating an organisationally secure environment, meaning that staff understand the extent and limits of their own and each others' roles and are able to function within them. This is likely to prevent conflicts between staff which may give rise to confusion and uncertainty among those for whom they care.

We should also recognise the ability of a manager to establish the kind of therapeutic milieu in which clinical nurses and midwives are able to provide genuinely helpful care for people who are grieving. In one maternity unit, I was told repeatedly about the admirable management skills of a midwife whose job was threatened due to the recent closure of a clinical area:

Yolandy We had a very good senior midwife up there, she really helped us a lot and helped us to cope a lot.

In view of their overwhelming perception of working under pressure, the need for managerial action to provide adequate numbers of appropriately skilled staff becomes even more important:

Molly Spending enough time listening to the mother can be difficult in these big wards. When you have 28 or 32 patients in the ward it can be, and you only have 4 staff.

Some of the midwives told me how they made decisions about the allocation of their own time and Gay recounted how she sought support from midwives in another area:

Gay Well, that lady that had the stillbirth, we were busy that day but I just stayed with her. Y'know and the rest of the patients I dealt with when the other staff came on. Y'know? I'm just going from that one experience that I had. I really stayed with her until she went down to the labour ward. She got priority. Yeah. And you can always ring to the labour ward – if they're quiet

– for help, which is quite good in this unit. If the place is quiet they'll come up and give you a helping hand.

I have been considering the role of the manager in providing support for individual midwives who feel stressed by the demands of their work and the limited resources available to them. These short-term managerial interventions provide much-needed on-the-spot support, but they have to be reinforced by more long-term, ongoing support which, in the same way, is likely to result from management innovation.

Group support and counselling services

In this section I look at the more formal organisation of support for staff caring for the mother who is grieving. I consider, first, the systems of group support which have been described and then move on to the counselling services which may or may not be available to staff.

There are three essential requirements of a staff support system (Bender & Swan-Parente, 1983):

(1) The opportunity for a member of staff who feels herself to be under stress to take 'time out'. This would involve her moving to a quiet space for a few 'reflective moments' to catch up on her thinking, which is all too easily overtaken by doing.
(2) A suitable forum where members of staff are able to articulate their feelings about recent events. A neutral and non-threatening environment is crucial for the effective functioning of this forum.
(3) The provision of time for members of staff to explore openly their feelings about their work.

Much of the literature about support groups describes them in terms of already having become established. This approach may be less than helpful if this form of group support does not exist, so I look, by way of introduction, at the way in which these groups may be developed.

In Southampton a member of the midwifery teaching staff involved a psychiatrist in establishing an informal, interdisciplinary support group (Roch, 1987). The group welcomed visitors, such as representatives from SANDS and other lay support groups, and bereaved mothers, to contribute. The author emphasises the non-hierarchical nature of this group. This lack of a hierarchical structure is clearly crucial if a support group is to provide the safe environment in which more reluctant colleagues are able to 'open up'. The organisers deserve credit for breaking through the hierarchical barriers, although unfortunately we are not told how this remarkable feat was achieved, as such structures are all too pervasive in midwifery.

Similarly, the multidisciplinary nature of this group appears to be another of its strengths. The membership included a range of personnel, some of whom were unrelated to the hospital or to nursing or midwifery. The reluctance of medical staff to become involved is clearly a source of regret to the organisers and we may question the reason for such reluctance.

In Preston a support group with a different remit was established (Sherratt, 1987). Interaction between lay people and professional carers is a priority for this group; consciousness-raising features as a major element – 'the topic needed to be brought to the notice of the general public'. The support of members of staff to parents appears to be secondary to providing information and help for grieving parents and those near to them. In spite of this, the passage of information is clearly a two-way exercise; this results in staff learning, from those who have actually experienced perinatal grief, of the most appropriate way to care.

An account of setting up a medical and nursing staff group in an NNU indicates some of the problems involved (Bender & Swan-Parente, 1983). Non-attendance was initially a problem, which the organisers solved by negotiation with nursing managers about the provision of suitable accommodation and time. Non-attendance may have been due to the lack of a safe environment and anxiety about the maintenance of personal defence systems. A generally acceptable format eventually evolved in which staff built on known case histories.

In the context of establishing a terminal care support team, Dunlop and Hockley (1990) explore the necessity for and pitfalls of organising an ongoing multidisciplinary support group. They describe how the initial 'honeymoon period' for the group was abruptly ended by the realisation of the enormity of the task and mismatches between needs and skills. The impact of having to constantly deal with death shocked some group members as did the perception of lack of support from 'uncooperative doctors, unfeeling nurses and ungrateful patients'.

The challenge of working as an effective team required facing up to personal and professional conflicts and overcoming the tendency to suppress them; the authors describe working through what they call 'chronic niceness', which was a short-term strategy to disguise inevitable ill-feelings. Several months of 'chronic niceness' were necessary before the group felt safe enough with each other to respect others' strengths and to give them credit in a non-paternalistic way.

These authors show us the value of group meetings for reflecting on difficult events. While working out 'what and who' made the situation difficult, allocating blame became a pitfall. Dunlop and Hockley go on to spell out the value of out-of-work group activities in helping to build relationships. Examples include pub lunches, theatre visits, picnics and other outings.

A major benefit of support groups lies in their ability to help us to work towards more realistic goals in our care of the dying (Osterweis *et* al., 1984). Our failure to meet unrealistic expectations may lead to withdrawal from involvement with patients, their relatives and colleagues. We may use a suitably safe and supportive group to ventilate our feelings of inadequacy. If we are able to deal with our negative feelings in this way, there are benefits not only for those for whom we care, but we, the carers, are likely to be more satisfied with the support we provide (Beszterczey, 1977).

In advocating peer support groups, Bond (1986) recognises the largely untapped ability of nurses to support each other. Referring to other non-peer support groups, she draws our attention to the willingness of 'group leaders', who tend to be male, to listen to the difficulties of a largely female caring staff. In contrast to this willingness to lead and listen, she highlights the reluctance of these leaders to relinquish their obviously responsible role by facilitating leadership skills within the group. Bond's accusation of such groups generating dependency among female colleagues may carry a familiar ring.

A problem which affects the organisation of support groups is the difficulty of making time. By definition, those of us who work in stressful environments are short of time. The question inevitably arises of how we, as individuals, are able to find time to give and receive support. Is it possible or appropriate for those of us who work in high-tech or otherwise stressful areas to assume that our employers will allow time for this form of recovery?

The problem of time was raised by Bender and Swan-Parente (1983) and also by Roch (1987). The solution Roch and her colleagues resorted to was to arrange the group sessions to be held during the changeover of shifts, when traditionally there has been an overlap resulting in an approximately two-hour period with a double staff complement. This 'overlap' has traditionally been used for a range of activities which some consider inessential, such as meetings or teaching, but it has now largely disappeared. The result is that alternative time slots now have to be identified.

The limited extent to which health authorities, health boards and trusts are prepared to make time available for support activities is raised by Cole (1993) in the context of group counselling. He shows us that the unpreparedness of employing authorities to allow support time reflects the limited priority given to staff welfare and perhaps, indirectly, to the support of those for whom we care.

It may be that Coles' suggestion of group counselling and support for those of us caring for people who are grieving is an ideal to aim for. Tschudin (1985) makes what may be a more realistic suggestion which comprises establishing services within an existing framework. She advocates that existing occupational health provision should extend its remit to include counselling services. She implicitly recognises the cost implications of providing this service when she states 'health authorities need to believe in the principle that prevention is better than cure'. Are staff support services another example of a phenomenon which is widely recommended, but rarely encountered?

A remembrance service

We all recognise the benefits of a funeral service for those who are grieving. I would like to question whether we, the caring staff, may appropriately use the funeral to express our grief, our support for the family and our support for each other? This concept emerged in my recent research project, initially in the context of the baptism of a still-born baby whose mother requested that Gay, the midwife, perform this rite. I asked Gay about her reaction to this request:

Gay   I suppose that the service does help the staff a bit. You do ... you probably do feel that you're doing something. I think the parents quite like it.

Ottily recounted her difficulty in going to the funeral:

Ottily   I've never attended a baby's funeral. I suppose I've chickened out from going.

On the other hand Zy was able to recount her very different experience:

Zy   I go down to the hospital chapel with them ... for the service. I think it is probably for both our sakes; not just for the parents, I think for the staff's sake as well, it makes a difference. I think of Jane, she is a staff midwife and not just newly qualified. She'd been so involved ... with the lady who had the stillbirth and she had a talk with her. And we arranged a service and Jane came down to the service with us and afterwards she said, 'I feel a lot better'. We laughed at that so I think it really does the staff good as well as the parents themselves.

Our presence at the funeral requires great sensitivity. If the family is still experiencing anger or if some blame is being allocated, we may not be welcome at an essentially family event.

Summary

In this chapter I have considered the problems which we, as members of staff, may encounter when caring for a mother who is grieving the loss of her baby. Using data collected during my recent research, I have shown some of the reasons why we find this situation so difficult. I have then moved on to discuss the solutions which have been suggested to help us to cope better, in the hope that we will be able to provide more effective care.

Chapter 10
Staff Grieving and Crying

The ways in which we, as members of staff, manifest our feelings at the loss of a baby vary hugely. While some of us feel comfortable showing our feelings, others may wish to, yet find themselves unable to be so open; yet another group may feel the need for a 'stiff upper lip' approach. Our manifestation of our reactions to loss may be changing because of increasing openness among staff. In this chapter I show that change has happened since Bourne (1979) stated that, even though staff are 'flung apart' by such a loss, some are able to show only 'aversion and silence'.

Crying as grieving

The concern of nurses and midwives about whether it is appropriate to show grief through tears is reflected in the increasing exposure of this topic in the nursing media. A number of midwives and nurses narrate experiences of sharing women's grief by the use of touch, physical comfort and tears (Darbyshire, 1992). These narratives imply the reluctance of others to 'get involved' by showing emotions. Each of the narratives concluded positively by indicating the benefits of sharing emotions for both the staff member and the woman or patient (Diekelmann, 1992; Walker, 1992).

Here I consider how staff feel about those occasions when they may have cried and the factors which affect whether or not they cry. As well as using the limited literature on this topic, I draw on the comments made by midwives during my recent study of the care of mothers who do not have their babies with them (Mander, 1992d).

The reluctance of midwives to acknowledge that they have cried with a mother, implied in Darbyshire's narratives (1992), is apparent in Nancy's account of her care of a mother relinquishing her baby for adoption:

Nancy I went with her to see her baby and she spoke to the baby and told her baby how she was sorry about giving him up and just explained that she couldn't look after him. It was really nice for someone who had denied it for so long . . .

Author   How did you manage?

Nancy   I was OK . . . and . . . no, I was crying actually.

The uncertainty many midwives feel about crying, which becomes clearer in the interviews described later, emerges in Marie's slightly defensive account of her more long-term relationship with the mother of a dying baby:

Marie   There was a woman we had in . . . whose baby eventually died at three months. We became very close and very supportive to that mother and when her baby died we were all upset and we were crying along with the mother.

Author   Was that OK?

Marie   We were crying, but that did not affect our ability to care. Even though we were upset we were still able to do our jobs. The day I don't shed a tear over a dead baby is the day I walk out the door of this place.

That we experience ambivalence about showing emotions to those for whom we care is clear and will become clearer. The mother's need for emotional contact with the midwife is apparent in the comment of a mother relinquishing her son for adoption:

Ursula   After I came home . . . and the midwife came to see me, she was really lovely. When she was making her last visit she put her arm round me and gave me a big hug. It meant so much to me and it was so different from others I had met.

Describing how nurses may experience and show their sorrow, Bond (1986) discusses patients' appreciation of such a 'spontaneous demonstration of empathy' and the benefits for the patient, who may then be in a better position to deal with their own pain.

Crying and helping

The midwives I interviewed interpreted their preparedness to cry with a bereaved mother in terms of sharing emotions, or perhaps the potential for common feelings.

Joy   It's not out of the ordinary but I often find myself crying with them. This is because I hurt for them – it could be me.

Polly   Yes, I have had tears in my eyes many a time with them, it is just a natural thing I think. Just talking about it, it is natural to sympathise with them. I think it's human and what they need is the human touch.

Florrie   Well y'know everybody is human . . . what would be wrong, y'know, for somebody to feel a lump in their throat and start crying? I think that is quite acceptable, and just to show that you have got feelings as well – and care.

The midwife's powerful sense of identification with the mother is obvious in these comments. Shared values and common experience are crucial in many aspects of midwives' care. They told me that they draw on many sources of knowledge and information when they are deciding on how to care, but the significance of their personal and occupational experience cannot be overstated (Mander, 1992b).

The naturalness and lack of deliberation when midwives cry seems to matter to those I interviewed. Even though it is spontaneous to behave in this open way, we don't always find it easy or comfortable.

Fanny   I personally can get quite emotional with the mother. Like if she was crying and talking, I could very easily join in and show that I also feel for her. That can help if she knows that you genuinely have sympathy with them and it's not just your job.

Author   How do you feel about that?

Fanny   I wouldn't say I feel comfortable, no. I have done it. I mean if I do genuinely feel if I was upset with someone I do genuinely feel that way. I wouldn't just do it to try to make them feel better. With someone losing their baby it's a very emotional thing for us, just as well as the mother. I certainly wouldn't be afraid to let someone know I felt sympathy and be upset at what had happened. I wouldn't be afraid to do that.

Fanny's comments introduce the spectre of the sense of failure which may be encountered by those of us who work in the maternity area, as well as the possibility of the reappearance of memories of other losses which may constitute 'unfinished business'.

Disapproving

As well as crying exposing the humanity and hence the vulnerability of us all, there are additional dimensions which we must consider when nurses and midwives contemplate crying. A midwife recounting her care of a mother adjusting to her newborn son's terminal illness illustrates some of these dimensions (Walker, 1992):

We cried together. I apologised for crying; I tried to say how unprofessional it was and that I was trained not to break down.

This quotation raises two of the significant issues in the context of staff crying. These are:

- the concept of 'professionalism'
- the education or training which prepares nurses and midwives to behave professionally.

It is necessary to assume that the term 'professional' in this context is being used to mean efficient and distant rather than any other professional characteristics. Darbyshire's commentary on Walker's narrative takes up the use of the term 'professional', suggesting that when used in this way, the concept is so 'perverse' as to be unrelated to any form of human experience. The 'perversity' of this term does not prevent it from being widely used, perhaps as a coping mechanism (Menzies, 1961):

Bessie   There are really two schools of thought about [crying]. First, there is the old school which says that you must retain your professional thing quite intact. The second view is that you grieve with the woman. I think that it really depends on the midwife and the woman. I am quite happy to hold her hand or to put my arm round her shoulder, but I think that you need to stay a professional.

The midwives were well-aware that their behaviour in crying with grieving parents might engender disapproval:

Emily   I know some people think that it is not professional, but I do sometimes cry with the mother as this lets her see that we are human.
Ottily   You can have a little cry . . . and nobody thinks any the less of you. You never used to be able to do that.
Queeny   Yes, I have cried with a woman who has lost her baby. I think that you should be able to, after all it is a human thing to do and we are all human. I know that some people think that nurses should not cry, but I think that is wrong. We need to be able to share [her] sorrow.

The fear may exist that the perceived disapproval may actually materialise into overt criticism, so that, at a time when we expect helpful support from our colleagues, we may render ourselves even more vulnerable to hostile criticism:

Queeny   There was a [mother] recently who lost her baby. I was very upset about it and so I cried with her. . . . I had to go to see the Nursing Officer about something and she said to me, 'What are you so upset for?' Some people don't approve.

Disapproval of crying was highlighted by Dunlop and Hockley (1990) in the context of nursing dying adults. These authors discuss the benefits of maintaining a 'calm demeanour' as opposed to the suppression of 'strong emotions'. They show us the role of nurse training in creating the 'pull yourself together' ethos.

Similarly, Walker's quotation leads me to question the appropriateness of midwifery and nursing education which teaches not only effective coping, but also maintenance of a veneer of efficiency:

Kerrie   . . . but you know obviously you've got be very careful to keep your emotions in check . . . you feel very close to tears . . . you can feel the tears springing into your eyes but . . . y'know. I don't know why. I think it is something that is drummed into you during your training or that with upsetting things you've got to put on this brave face and, you know, just show the patient that you are coping and that you can't burst into tears.

A nursing student's harrowing account of observing and learning from others about coping with the death of a pre-term baby illustrates that better qualified and more experienced colleagues may have equal difficulty (Anon, 1993b).

Although it is clear that midwives consider that crying may sometimes be appropriate, they are both aware and wary of the possibility of disapproval by other members of staff. Inevitably, the openness which sharing grief requires also renders the carer more vulnerable to criticism.

Crying real tears

While we may be generally approving of midwives crying with grieving parents, the implications of this approval for our midwifery practice may be less direct. For some of us there is no difficulty in putting our ideas about crying into practice:

Joy   For me it's so easy, so natural to put my arms around her and to cry with her. I often have.

For other midwives, such as Deidre, while approving of the idea of a midwife crying, there may be a barrier to putting it into practice:

Deidre   If you feel like crying, I don't think you should stop yourself. I think some staff would probably not be able to cry in that situation because it wouldn't be comfortable. If that is the case, you have just got to be yourself. I haven't cried openly. I think I have had tears in my eyes and a lump in my throat, but I haven't actually sat down and cried.
Author   Is this because crying may affect your ability to care?
Deidre   I don't think that is true. I think if you are feeling like crying [and do] then you won't function any worse than if you bottle it up.
Hattie   I think if she's feeling strong emotions, I don't see that there's any crime if she does [cry]. I know it was maybe the old idea that we should remain detached from parents. I think we've been part of something very dramatic in the woman's life, we can't alter that.
Author   Have you [cried]?
Hattie   Well, maybe not cried in front of the patient but I have felt very, very sad, maybe have gone out . . . , felt very devastated if something has happened.

These quotations lead to the conclusion that we may actually find crying with the grieving mother to be less acceptable and hence less likely to happen than the recommendations of openness would suggest.

Places to cry

While a carer may feel uncomfortable sharing her tears with the grieving mother, she may still consider it appropriate to give expression to her emotions in a safe environment. I consider now where this safe place to vent emotions may be.

The traditional place in a hospital ward for the disposal of waste is the sluice. In the sluice, dirty linen is collected for transfer to the laundry, human waste is despatched, such as bedpans' contents, and used dressings are bagged ready for incineration. Although I, and possibly others, have used the sluice for the secret disposal of emotional waste, including fury, frustration and sorrow, it was not mentioned by any of the midwives. Similarly, the linen cupboard, often publicised as the location of various unmentionable activities (Bond, 1986), was not suggested as a suitable place for crying.

Although Zy was initially unable to admit to crying with the parents, she eventually recalled that she had used the changing room for her tears and that this prepared her to share their grief more openly:

Zy   I have probably not been actually in tears . . . I tell a lie, there is one time I was absolutely ... I had to adjourn into the changing room. I had got quite involved with one of the [mothers] . . . and I just burst into tears and I felt better after it, but I think possibly we'd got more involved than we normally do . . . I had to go back and see them, and they said, 'Oh, you've been crying'. So I had a chat with them, and a wee bubble again, and now I say it's OK. I think it does both parties good.

The staff room was also suggested as a suitable place for tears; for Ottily this was where she found emotional support from her colleagues:

Ottily   We all help and support each other when these things happen. You can have a little cry in the coffee room.

The emotional sustenance suggested by Ottily was also mentioned by Florrie in the form of liquid refreshment, but this was more in the context of providing a route by which she could remove herself from the presence of the grieving mother:

Florrie   I think it's OK [to cry]. . . . Although she should not cry to the point of breaking down, maybe go out of the room, maybe have a cup of tea in between, maybe go out and do other jobs.

Kerrie's attempts to remove herself from the grieving parents appear to have actually served to open up the communication between her and the parents:

Kerrie   You can't burst into tears and you just have to ... as I say, sometimes they come outside the door and there you are having a wee cry to yourself and then you all go back in ..., y'know.

I have suggested that the sluice may be the appropriate place for crying in view of its function of disposing of waste. The midwives lead me to believe that crying is a more constructive activity than just disposing of waste, akin to finding sustenance, as in the coffee room. This may also be applied to the comments made by Zy, whose use of the changing room for crying helped to prepare her for a more open relationship with the parents. This more constructive interpretation of crying is also found in an account by a poorly-supported student nurse caring for a dying child (Anon, 1993a), who found herself in tears in the ward kitchen, the place for preparing nourishment.

Control

The literature and my research show that some degree of ambivalence towards crying openly still exists among midwives and nurses. Although generally accepting of crying with a grieving mother, the midwives I interviewed invariably expressed some concern about limiting or controlling their need to cry. It may be that these midwives' underlying concerns about the acceptability of crying, learned through midwifery and nurse training and years of practice, manifested themselves in the need to control this quintessentially uncontrollable act:

Hilary   I've been near to tears a couple of times ... But you can't get too involved, you have got to have a cut-off point or else you wouldn't be able to handle it.

This cut-off point is a recurring theme in midwives' accounts of the extent to which they allow themselves to cry. Effie mentions the self-awareness which is necessary if this self-imposed cut-off point is to operate:

Effie   I think it is fair enough for you to be grieving along with her as long as you are in control of the situation ... I think it may be quite a good thing for [the mother] that someone is there sharing the grief, so long as they are aware of what they are doing themselves. I think there is a situation where you can be upset along with someone but still remain professional.

As midwives we identify our own cut-off points, beyond which we fear being unable to function. The midwives spelt out the importance of identifying this point in terms of fear of going too far:

Irene I have cried many times. I don't totally break down, you really must keep control of the situation, but I would certainly shed a tear or two.

Kay It's a very sad experience. And you should show them that you actually care and that it's not something that you do seven days of the week ... I think there's crying and crying and there's a few tears and having the screaming abdabs, and you're no use to anybody if you're like that.

Annie I must admit I am quite an emotional person myself and obviously you don't want to get hysterical or anything like that. I'll be quite honest – I can't help myself shedding a few tears. You just have to make it very quiet and discrete ... You don't want them having to feel sorry for you, which would obviously be totally inappropriate ...

These comments by Kay and Annie show that their cut-off point has been fixed to prevent their crying causing their presence to be either unhelpful or counter-productive. The point identified by Annie was widely accepted among the midwives as the cut-off point, that is when the parents need to support the midwife.

Another criterion which the midwives use to help them to identify their own cut-off points was their ability to function effectively. This may be similar to the 'professionalism' already discussed, but some explained this concept in more helpful terms:

Ottily You can always cry with the couple. I think that the important thing is for you to be strong in order to be able to help them.

Leonie Sometimes it can be very draining on yourself emotionally, but the point at which you become no help to her is the point where it completely overtakes you. When you can't come into the room without getting terribly upset and being so upset, probably upsetting them further. We're in danger of that if we are not recognising that that is possible.

This point emphasises our need for the self-awareness mentioned already by Effie and commended by Cathcart (1989). Leonie built on her ideas about self-awareness by describing her impression of midwives' need for clearly-defined personal limits:

Leonie I think there has to be [limits], we have to know where they are, and maybe if we are getting to that stage or feel it's getting too much then we have to stop short because then we stop being any help. We stop being the pillar of support that the mother so desperately needs.

Kay The last thing the mother needs is to be comforting somebody who is supposed to be helping her. But I don't think that a moist eye or a tear running down my cheek is going to do her any harm. Obviously if you feel that it's upsetting her then that is the time to withdraw, and just leave them on their own and get yourself together.

The midwife having to withdraw from caring is something we have to consider if her ability to provide care is likely to be compromised by her emotional reaction to the mother's loss.

> *Leonie*   Maybe she can take time out ... if there are two midwives then it's easier ... the midwife then needs to go and talk it over with one of her fellow colleagues, get out her emotions about it ... she can't bottle it up herself or I think she'd probably go off feeling very depressed and maybe not handle the next one quite so well...

The possibility of the midwife's emotional response causing her to withdraw from a grieving situation obviously has management and staffing implications, as well as the personal aspects already mentioned. Emotional factors are one of the areas which midwives need to take into account when planning their work at the beginning of a shift:

> *Leonie*   If she feels that when the staff are allocated that this is a situation which at this particular time she feels she couldn't quite handle, she could say, 'I prefer not to look after this lady because I don't feel that I might be as supportive as somebody else might be given different circumstances'. This would apply if she was feeling more susceptible for some reason, there may be some background upset in her own life, there might have been a death of any member in the family, then she's less likely ..., maybe she will understand but be less likely to be emotionally supportive, and more likely to feel the greater emotion herself, I don't know. She may be less able to give because she's still handling this experience, a similar experience, herself and maybe hasn't come to terms with it enough in order to help this particular couple.

The need for the midwife to be in control of her crying emerged strongly, as did the anxiety that crying might impair the midwife's functioning. This need to assume control over her behaviour may appear to contrast sharply with the midwife's wish to behave in a spontaneous or natural way when sharing the woman's grief. I suggest that this contrast is not real, as we need certain boundaries within which to operate if we are to allow ourselves to behave in a natural and human way.

Inability to cry

I have already touched on some of the management implications of the midwife sharing the mother's grief. These factors apply mainly in the labour ward setting, where one midwife would be caring for one grieving mother or couple. This emphasis is not inappropriate in view of the fact that, because of the likelihood of early transfer home, the labour ward is where a grieving mother spends most of her hospital stay.

In the postnatal ward the demands on the midwife's time are likely to be different, in that she may be caring less intensively, but for a larger number of mothers. If one of those mothers is grieving the loss of her baby, the midwife may encounter difficulties with the constant adjustment and readjustment between mothers in differing emotional states:

Carrie   You have got to deal with this one woman, often due to staff allocations and the 'busyness' of the ward; not only are you looking after this one grieving mother, partner, siblings, what have you, you've got to be next door with somebody who has had a nice bouncing baby and be happy for that person. It can be quite difficult sometimes to really have a chance to – or feel that you can – really express your feelings. A lot of the time it is so sad, all you want to do is to start crying for the woman and then you have to come out of the door and start coping with the rest of the ward and be seen to be in command. It can be difficult.

This is clearly not just a short-term problem involving the midwife making adjustments between very different situations in which mothers' needs vary hugely. The longer-term implications for midwives of being prevented from expressing their feelings during the on-duty period need attention. This scenario places an intolerable strain on the informal support network, which may have lasting effects on midwives and those to whom they are close.

Carrie's inability to cry is comparable to the difficulties recounted by a junior house officer, whose experience of her father's death leads Martin (1993) to plead for a more human medical stereotype. She describes her 'horrendous hours, storing up the pain [of grief] until it erupts in a flood of exhausted irritability when I come off duty'. In this description we see some aspects in common with Carrie. Martin clearly spells out the adverse effects of her on-duty stress on her off-duty support network, which are likely to be similar for other carers.

Martin's search for insights into medical practitioners' difficulties is illuminated in a philosophical paper by Adshead and Dickenson (1993). These writers probe the reasons for the 'contrasting approaches' taken by 'doctors and nurses' in the care of people who are dying. Whereas Martin refers to the medical practice of using science as a shield from reality, presumably another example of the defence mechanisms already mentioned, Adshead and Dickenson discuss medical reliance on the positivistic medical model, which involves denying values and beliefs a place in science. These writers commend the more broadly-based system of nursing education and the more heterogeneous population from which nursing students originate, implying a breadth of experience denied to our medical colleagues.

In her paper, Martin regrets the 'outmoded macho image of invulnerability' still prevalent among her peers. Likewise, Adshead and Dickenson identify a 'cult of macho toughness' imbued during medical training, which is particularly stringent for female students. This issue becomes most poignant at the point where Martin, regretting her inability by virtue of her medical background to grieve openly, observes 'were I a nurse, a few tears would be permissable'.

Adshead and Dickenson interpret Martin's observation in terms of the broad gender differences between nurses and medical practitioners; the tendency to tears being more stereotypically female in western societies, allowing nurses to cry. It may be appropriate to question whether female nurses and midwives have assimilated the more masculine attitudes of medical colleagues to this behaviour, in the same way as they have assimilated other medical concepts (Pearson & Vaughan, 1989).

By way of contrast, in her case study of a mother whose first child died in the neonatal period, Littlewood (1992) commends the helpful support that medical staff were able to provide around the time of her bereavement. This account culminates in a simple statement which may reflect changing medical attitudes: The paediatrician who attended the baby wept with the parents when the child died.

It is necessary to question whether the permissability of tears for female nurses observed by Martin might relate to an imbalance in the power relationship between client and carer. If this applies, a more equal or balanced relationship between 'professionals' and those they care for would reduce perceptions of vulnerability to allow openness in sharing grief. The data I have drawn on indicate midwives' perceptions of partnership with those for whom they care, with a few nagging doubts about professionalism.

Summary

I have discussed only our outward signs of grief and have attempted neither to probe the feelings underlying these outward manifestations nor to describe the stress engendered among midwives and other staff caring for grieving mothers (see Chapter 9).

I have focused on the way in which crying helps staff members and the extent to which we consider that our tears facilitate the progress of the mother's grief. It appears that, generally, midwives feel that increasing openness in sharing feelings about the loss of a baby is beneficial. We should treat this statement cautiously; the limited literature on our medical colleagues' responses and the large proportion of personal accounts of crying written under pseudonyms and 'Anon' indicate that openness is still far from complete (Benjamin, 1993; Anon, 1993a; Anon, 1993b).

Chapter 11
The Role of Lay Support Groups

I became aware, during my research on mothers who do not have babies with them (Mander, 1992d), of the importance midwives attach to lay support groups' contribution to the care of a grieving mother. The benefits have been recognised in the literature on self-help in general; examples include research by Parkes (1980) and Raphael (1984b) focusing on widows, which showed the benefits of a secure social support network, including lay groups. There has, however, been little research on lay support for grieving parents.

In this chapter I look at the functioning of lay perinatal support groups, first, briefly considering what self-help involves; then, in order to apply this to perinatal bereavement, I employ as a framework the observations which midwives made during my recent study. Finally, I summarise the essential issues which arise in the care of the grieving mother.

I use the term 'lay support' to differentiate this care from that provided by health care providers, which is the primary focus of this book. The interface between the care which health care providers offer and that provided by others deserves attention because it is here that our care of the grieving mother may be found wanting.

Lay support systems include a more informal sector, the family and friends, which is highly individual, as well as the less informal sector on which I focus here. This more organised system of lay support comprises groups which are established to help the members deal or cope with a common problem, in this context perinatal grief. Self-help has been defined in terms of six features (Knight & Hayes, 1981):

- voluntary activity
- members having a common problem
- meeting for mutual benefit
- sharing the roles of helper and helped
- constructive action towards common goals
- groups being organised by members without external support.

Formerly known as 'mutual aid', self-help is known to many in the form of groups like Alcoholics Anonymous (Adams, 1990; Richardson & Goodman, 1983).

Background

While attempting to disentangle the twin concepts of self-care and self-help, Kickbusch (1989) outlines the recent development of self-help. Our growing interest in self-help resulted from the growth of medical sociology in the 1950s and 1960s which, in turn, was a response to increasing medical power. The balance of power in the traditional 'patient–physician' relationship has been questioned in the work of writers such as Illich (1976). The growth of self-help was fuelled by social movements, such as the women's movement, which exposed concerns about the 'medicalisation' of healthy processes, such as childbearing.

Kickbusch asserts that self-help became more firmly established with the consumerist ethos of the 1970s. During this decade mutual learning and support was preferred to more medical approaches. Our growing realisation that each of us is the expert when it comes to our own functioning carried connotations of self-control and empowerment, causing the power balance in health care interactions to change. The more equal inputs carry an aura of assertiveness, which may be seen by some as a threat to the traditional, one-sided arrangement of professional dominance and the medical model. Kickbusch compares the concurrent moves from a disease to a health orientation and from a medical to a self-help approach. These upheavals were recognised in the publication of a new community health care programme (WHO, 1983).

Since this recognition by WHO, self-help has assumed even greater significance in the UK. Adams (1990), using a social work perspective, shows how self-help has contributed to people assuming control over their circumstances, that is, their empowerment. He, like Kickbusch, emphasises that this assumption of control carries the inevitable implication that control must be relinquished by another group. Obviously, those relinquishing power are the professional carers; this change in the balance of power may not only be threatening to professionals (Lindenfield & Adams, 1984) but is likely to 'complicate' or damage the relationship between the consumer, client or patient and their formal carer. That self-help usually evolves to satisfy needs left unmet by deficiencies or gaps in formal provision does little to alleviate feelings of threat.

These anxieties or uncertainties about the benefits of self-help are answered in the work of Humble and Unell (1989), who explain the difficulty some people have in understanding this concept. They discuss the marginality of self-help, which many regard as a 'fringe activity' or a 'harmless diversion . . . which can usually be safely ignored'.

The difficulty of understanding the concept is aggravated by the limited durability of self-help groups, the diversity of the problems addressed and the multiplicity of members' expectations. Our inability to 'pigeon-hole' self-help into traditional health care models clearly does not facilitate understanding.

The functions of self-help groups are similarly vulnerable to mis-understanding and unrealistic expectations, which is a major reason for the demise of potentially effective self-help groups (Miller & Webb, 1988). Members' knowledge of the basic functions of a self-help group (Lindenfield & Adams, 1984) would help ensure a common purpose, including:

- reduction of isolation
- facilitating problem solving
- providing coping skills
- identifying other sources of help
- improving confidence
- empowering people to improve their own lives
- giving emotional support
- providing an alternative to medication
- organising social contacts
- undertaking pressure group activities and publicity.

Self-help in the context of perinatal grief

When asked about the support available for the grieving mother, the midwives I interviewed mentioned professional, family and other lay support. Here I relate the midwives' comments to the literature on self-help in both general situations and in the context of perinatal grief (Mallinson, 1989).

Benefiting

The midwives were generally confident that the grieving mother would benefit from contact with a mother who had experienced a similar loss and also through being involved with a support group:

Author　What would you say is the aim of midwives' care for this mother?
Queeny　... You can tell them about SANDS; I think the contact with other bereaved mothers is helpful.
Irene　... In terms of the long-term care of this mother, we are able to put her in touch with societies formed by mothers who have experienced a similar problem. There are support groups that would be able to help her or it may be possible to put her into contact directly with a mother I know who has been through a similar experience. I think that they are helpful to this mother.

> *Lucy*   ... I think there are a lot of other methods of support that we have to give her as well. Sometimes that can be just sitting talking to her, other times it can take the form of actual support groups that are available for women in these circumstances. We would give them advice, or there are Sisters working in the paediatric department – if her baby has been in the paediatric department – then they would be able to deal with all the different support groups that may be applicable to that person.

Making contact

Establishing contact with others in a similar situation is the first step in the 'self-help process' (Adams, 1990). He describes joining an established group or, alternatively, identifying with a like-minded person the need to initiate a new group. Either way, an essential precursor is the realisation that a problem exists and that with the help of others it may be manageable. *Passing on information* to a grieving mother about local groups was clearly seen as part of midwifery care:

> *Izzy*   I have, though, referred people to SANDS organisation. We have their telephone number in the ward. And I give her the telephone number before she goes.
> *Betty*   I think it is useful to put the bereaved mother in touch with a contact person [for a support group] before she is discharged.

The research project by Richardson and Goodman (1983) suggests that health care providers play an almost negligible role in providing information about local groups. Their intensive study of four self-help organisations (Mencap, Gingerbread, National Association of Widows and National Council for the Single Woman and her Dependants) showed that a large majority of new members were recruited by word of mouth and that publicity in print came a close second. Like Adams, these authors emphasise the need to overcome the psychological barrier of denial of the problem before help is sought. Richardson and Goodman suggest that stigma may make this hurdle quite insuperable, but the extent to which this applies in the context of perinatal grief is uncertain.

Being caught in a trap is how a grieving mother feels when she is ready and needing to talk about her grief but the midwife has stopped visiting and her partner has returned to work. In this situation a support group plays an important role:

> *Gay*   She felt she could've had somebody else to talk to. And she said that by the time she was ready to talk about it, there was nobody coming in to see her, y'know. And that was hard for her. Yeah, a self-help group probably would help, yes. And then it's trying to encourage a person to actually go and phone. They think they will probably cause a nuisance. Yeah, I think they would help.

Feelings of being trapped may be aggravated by the grieving mother's difficulty in preparing herself physically and psychologically to make the first move.

Making an out-of-the-blue approach to begin a relationship is especially daunting when a mother's grief makes her isolated and vulnerable. Richardson and Goodman (1983) described the 'hesitancy' among would-be joiners which they attribute to 'fear of the unknown' or 'lack of confidence'. These researchers focused on people who were either less vulnerable or whose problem was more common than grieving mothers, such as single parents; their sample experienced little difficulty in making this initial contact.

Penson (1990) details the 'emotional energy' necessary for a bereaved woman to make this first move and how she may 'put off telephoning for several days'. Are we able to help ease this first painful and tentative step?

Amy Another thing that you can do is guide them towards SANDS, and explain to them what it is and that if they need help they can get in touch with them or we can get in touch with them for them. Y'know . . . like breaking the ice.

Thus, some midwives tried to make that difficult first move. It is impossible to judge whether her helpfulness was successful or whether the mother's anxiety was simply moved a stage further along in the joining process.

Caution was expressed by some midwives, although almost all of them spoke positively about self-help groups. These midwives felt that some mothers would not be helped by these groups, either because of the nature of the group or the characteristics of the mother they would recommend to join it:

Shirley They can be very helpful. I think an awful lot depends on how well she has been counselled and how much help she needs. Some people do need the extra help and the support of outsiders. Some people would resent outsiders knowing what they would term 'their business'. They would term it interference. You've got to take it very carefully. You've got to decide – I have given out these addresses of self-help groups to mothers, but there are other odd mothers I have never approached with it because I know they wouldn't take to it.

Shirley was unable to explain the characteristics in a mother that would make her decide not to give this information. A very experienced midwife, having worked with mothers and babies for over 30 years, Shirley drew on empathy, intuition and gut feeling for many of her care decisions, including this one. Health care providers are clearly able to help mothers learn about support groups, although feelings about who would *want* to join such a group influence whether information is given.

Joining and not joining

The variation in the nature and organisation of self-help groups means that the concept of membership may not always be relevant (Robinson & Henry, 1977), but becoming part of the group is not possible until the person has at least attended a meeting. Like Shirley, some midwives emphasised the voluntary nature of support groups and the possibility that some mothers would not be keen to become involved.

Dorothy   They've got support groups for them, some of them like to have phone numbers and some of them aren't the least bit interested. They've got them if they need it.

Ginnie   I think it is a voluntary thing for the patient and her partner; if they want to contact SANDS they can.

Trudy   I think they have a role to play . . . I think it is the ultimate role often . . . I think it has a role and I think if the individual is wanting to go, that's great.

A common *criticism* of self-help is highlighted by Adams (1990), which may explain the reluctance of some people to join groups. He relates modern self-help to the bourgeois, paternalistic, charitable movements of the Victorian era and links the two phenomena by social class, claiming that self-help 'has often reflected the values of middle-class society'.

Adams' contention contrasts with the view that self-help originated with the trade unions (Miller & Webb, 1988) and, hence, is a working class concept. In their research examining the functioning of a range of self-help organisations, Miller and Webb (1988) distinguished social class influences. They found that those groups that focused on a single issue and that were affiliated to a national parent group showed a definite middle-class bias. On the other hand, non-affiliated groups which became established in urban areas tended to be more generalist and have a more working-class membership.

The observation of a middle-class tendency in the membership of national organisations is endorsed by the data of Richardson and Goodman (1983). The membership of four national organisations included a clear majority of non-manual workers (67.5%). Fear of a different value system may discourage a mother from attending in the first place or from returning to a group.

On the basis of their study, Richardson and Goodman conclude that the reasons for people not joining support groups may relate, first, to the lack of a suitable group or ignorance of its existence. Second, a person may decide not to join, either because they have the help they need, or because they fear being unwelcome or out of place.

Her *misgivings* at the prospect of joining a support group are recounted by a widowed psychotherapist (Rose, 1990). Categorising herself as an elitist non-joiner, she contemplates the value of support to groups of people to which she *definitely* does not belong, such as 'alcoholics and lost souls'. Her professional self distanced her by reminding her that she was 'the therapist, not the patient'.

Rose (1990) describes her fear of loss of uniqueness which group membership would bring, in that she was unprepared to recognise that others may have a similar experience. She eventually realised that her defences had protected her well in the early stages of her grief, but were in danger of isolating her and aggravating her sorrow. Rose had particular difficulty with the idea that she needed the help of a group, but managed to resolve her aversion to the benefit of herself and the group.

Penson (1990) suggests that a bereaved person may not wish to attend or join due to fear of a 'morbid' atmosphere, when the only common factor is the death of someone close. Alternatively, knowing that self-disclosure is a feature of support groups, some people may feel unready to discuss their experience. As a way of dealing with the fear mentioned by Penson, Lindenfield and Adams (1984) describe how new members may be helped to 'open up' in a less threatening way. They also explain the importance of group activities which are less grief-related, such as 'increasing togetherness' and, perhaps to counter fears of a morbid atmosphere, 'having fun'.

A successful support group has certain characteristics which make people comfortable attending it. These characteristics appear to be relevant to a perinatal support group and include the person feeling that (Miller & Webb, 1988):

- there is space for them there
- that there is a peer group for contact and friendship
- the group identity is congruent with the person's self-identity
- the group builds up members' self-esteem and confidence
- the group balances meeting members' needs with encouraging independence

Being in a crisis

Yolandy all of a sudden they're faced with a situation they can't cope with and it's something they've got to get used to, and it's easier if they can talk to somebody else who has been through the same situation. Reassuring for them as well, because I think a lot of the ladies get very frightened and the reactions they're having to the situation that they find themselves in. They're going through the grieving process. A lot of these young girls have never known bereavement in a family situation.

Although she did not mention the word, Yolandy's account of the grieving mother's feelings, brings to mind both the lay and the more psychologically-orientated concept of a crisis. The suddenness of the event is combined with the unexpected inability to cope with it, reminiscent of Caplan's definition (1961): A crisis is provoked when a person faces an obstacle to important life goals that is, for a time, insurmountable through customary methods of problem-solving.

Murgatroyd and Woolfe (1982) in their work on coping with crises consider the role of mutual aid, help and support. Their ideas on community self-help are of particular relevance to our support of the grieving mother because they advocate that helpers should encourage those in crisis to recognise the reality of their situation. The identification of the person's own strengths has much in common with the self-help ethos, as does the final outcome – independent functioning.

A more mundane view of crisis and the self-help response is presented by Robinson and Henry (1977). Accepting the increasingly finite resources of the formal care sector, they observe the absence of help when people most need it, or the difficulty of making an urgent appointment. This is contrasted with the availability of self-help contacts, whose experience of similar problems means that help is accessible immediately and freely. Many groups take the provision of direct help a stage further by encouraging the perception of being supported and by offering help before it has been sought.

Self-help and the health care system

The direct help offered by self-care groups, in contrast with the limited resources of the health care system, provides us with an example of how self-help and formal health care interact.

The *overlap* between support groups' help and formal care provision emerged in the midwives' comments. They were aware of the lack of resources, and considered that support groups would be able to fill the gap. To this extent they regarded the self-help groups as complementary to the formal services:

> *Ginnie*   I think you have to be very understanding . . . and you have to accept the fact that, should they require more counselling than you can actually give them, you must be ready to hand over care of these patients to SANDS or such a group of people.

Likewise, the relative inadequacy of statutory provision was recognised by 'officials', who envied the lack of bureaucracy and the immediacy of response in self-help groups (Richardson & Goodman, 1983). Despite this, these authors concluded that the role of self-help is to supplement formal care, as the consumers in their sample utilised professional help, by consulting 'various medical experts, social workers and advice officers'. They used self-help groups for mutual support or when needing the understanding of someone who had personal experience of a situation, leading to the authors' claim that self-help's reciprocity is its unique strength.

> *Wendy*   There are other people there you can talk to who've been through the same experience. They really understand. I've heard on one occasion the comment that [the staff] 'were so nice and tried to be so understanding but they really don't know how I feel' and I think that having places like SANDS they are talking to people who really do know what they are feeling and who have been through it themselves, that's bound to help . . .

The supplementary nature of self-help also emerged:

> *Trudy*   I think there is an awful lot more that could be done. I don't think we should just say . . . 'Here's the baby's registration, funeral bits and here are the self-help organisations . . .' Not that it does in reality actually happen like that, but I still think . . . there's more . . .

It is clear from the midwives' that they regard self-help as an important adjunct to their care, to the extent that it provides more extensive and longer-term care than they are able to offer, a partnership which is earnestly sought in the social work field (Richardson & Goodman, 1983). It is possible, however, for the implications of this 'partnership' to be interpreted less benignly, in that the spectre of manipulation by a dominant occupation arises (Lindenfield & Adams, 1984). Self-help may be used as a political football to justify cutbacks in statutory services or to encourage self-sufficiency (Adams, 1990).

Lack of groups

Examining the data and the literature on support groups brings me to consider resources, as raised by Betty in response to my open question:

> *Author*   What changes do you think are needed in the care of this mother?
> *Betty*   More bereavement support groups would be helpful.

Ginnie also observed the shortage of this form of care and was able to deduce both the immediate and underlying reasons:

> *Ginnie*   . . . unfortunately they don't seem to have enough . . . of them. We have a list of contacts but obviously if these ladies have other family they stop working for SANDS because of their own reasons, but I think it is like everything else, they are really underfunded.

Limited provision is similarly observed and regretted by Leon (1990), who considers that a dearth of counselling services exists in all areas of bereavement support, despite its value being well-established by research.

Reciprocal helping

I have already mentioned that mutual support based on common experience, or reciprocity, is the unique strength of self-help; but whether someone experiencing difficulty is best placed to support others in the same situation is questionable. Richardson and Goodman (1983) argue that a person struggling to manage her own life may lack the emotional energy to support another.

Their criticism is answered by the concept of 'serial reciprocity' being fundamental to self-help. This involves those for whom a longer time has elapsed from their experience being better able to support those who are newly afflicted. Thus, the people who attend group meetings may initially do so because they hope to receive support, information, direct help or social contacts. As they become more confident within the group and their problem resolves, they find themselves able to give more. This may be in the form of advice and support to relatively new members or as a commitment to organising the group.

A midwife explained this concept:

Irene . . . peoples' roles may be reversed; the bereaved couple having been helped may better find that they are able to help others in a similar situation. The group may not be of any help immediately after the birth, but she may be the sort of woman who wants to grieve alone and then maybe contact such a group later when she is ready to. She may find that she is better able to give support at that stage to other women who have lost their babies, rather than being the one who accepts others' support.

Irene distinguishes women who benefit once or twice from belonging to a group. The twice-benefiting woman is supported initially and later gains satisfaction from supporting others; whereas another woman may benefit only once, on the later occasion.

Whereas Irene presents serial reciprocity as a dichotomy, Klass (1985) views it as a continuum comparable with grieving. At one end of the continuum the mother is immersed in her grief and able only to accept support, but as her grieving progresses she needs less support and is able to give more. She eventually reaches the opposite end of the continuum when her grief is resolved and her support needs have diminished. At this point she has a wealth of experience of both grieving and being supported, enabling her to help others.

Hospital-based support groups

I have been emphasising the *mutuality* of support through self-help, in that shared experience underpins empathy. The extent to which professional carers, who have not shared this experience, are able to facilitate group support now deserves attention. The midwives I interviewed did not claim that hospital-based support groups were self-help groups, but their existence leads us to think about the input of the formal carers:

Deidre Special Care has got parents' support groups and things. They don't have a counsellor but they do have groups.

Hilary There is a society in this unit for parents who have been bereaved. It is run by two of the sisters and each bereaved mother is sent a personal invitation to ask her to come along to the group which meets monthly in the hospital.

A bereavement group

Following Gohlish's (1985) research a bereavement group was set up in the maternity unit (Tom-Johnson, 1990). The role of the carers in initiating the group and inviting bereaved mothers is described and comparisons are made with SANDS and TAMBA. The feedback provided by the group has led to many improvements in care. The nature of the carers' ongoing involvement in this group is unclear, though Tom-Johnson states that carers are present to answer parents' questions about, for example, future pregnancies.

Pitfalls

The pitfalls for professionals in these groups, discussed by Klass and Shinners (1983), warn us that we should limit our natural inclination to provide detailed factual information and arrange referrals. Lavoie (1982, cited in Gartner & Reissman, 1984) also recommends that we should avoid recourse to purely professional knowledge and certainly not regard it as our only expertise. This cautious approach aims to prevent 'professionalising the group', in which we (not the members) become the primary source of knowledge. Clearly such an intervention would endanger the mutuality of the group and totally alter the form of interaction.

Establishment

The development of a self-help bereavement support group by a nurse is detailed by Penson (1990). She explains how unique nursing skills may be used to found and establish the group, including finding a suitable venue, identifying potential members and creating a warm and encouraging atmosphere. Penson summarises the nurse's function as being facilitating contact between those who need help and those who can offer it. She then goes on to emphasise the need for the nurse to withdraw from the group, allowing it to continue to evolve as determined by the members. The professional may continue to be available to act as a troubleshooter in the event of problems such as internal rivalry or declining membership (Miller & Webb, 1988).

Difficulties

Adopting an unashamedly political orientation, Adams (1990) probes the difficulties which professionals are likely to encounter when, because of limited resources, the inevitable increase in self-help requires them to relinquish power to newly-empowered consumers. Such a realignment may give rise to feelings of threat among some professionals. Their difficulty may be due to the traditional view of self-help as 'at best wasteful of resources and at worst downright counterproductive' (Adams, 1990).

Although self-help is viewed positively by those I interviewed, there is a general element of caution, if not anxiety, underlying professional responses to it. This applies in spite of benefits which accrue for carers from groups' activities.

Helping the carers

A feature of self-help groups which was of importance to the midwives I interviewed but which does not appear in the general self-help literature relates to the assistance which they provide for carers. This may be in the form of information, which operated at two levels.

The first level is the provision of feedback on the care provided for the grieving mother:

Zy   I've been thinking about going along ... to find out what the women felt themselves about what we all did for them ... how we helped or what we can still do to help.
Bessie   The only thing ... was a reading list I got. I'm not sure where it came from, I think it might have been SANDS ... the talk by the people from SANDS also helped. I was able to get a lot of feedback about my care of these women through SANDS.

The need for mothers' views to inform our care, usually available through research, was raised by Tom-Johnson (1990).

The second level at which self-help groups assist midwives is in their information and literature and through formal and informal face-to-face contacts. Although the printed material is designed to be distributed to grieving mothers, it is not unreasonable that the carer should read the material first, if only to ensure that it is acceptable.

Ginnie I read the SANDS stuff that they have. It's very good literature that they hand out to the patients about various ... it's a question-and-answer type thing and its showing you questions that partners are asking and other people have asked and I've found that very helpful.

The gifts of equipment which self-help groups donate to maternity units serve to influence practice as well as support the staff:

Zy I think [groups] probably will be helpful, I know the lady, the contact that we have, that we got the Moses basket through; she's a very nice lady, and she's very helpful, even just for us to talk to ...

Hattie Oh, SANDS are good, very good, they have given us a book of remembrance which is very nice.

Tom-Johnson lists examples of items which may be donated in this way and she goes on to detail their value. Her examples include a book of remembrance and the folders in which grieving parents are able to keep their mementoes of their baby.

Problems

As mentioned already some midwives were cautious about recommending a grieving mother to attend a self-help group because the mother might not fit in with the group and might be hurt by the experience.

Dwelling on grief

The activities of the group being unhelpful also caused concern to some midwives:

Ruby There is a ... organisation called SANDS. I think they are very good. I think they do a lot of good. But some of them maybe go a little over the top, and get taken over by the kinds of women who focus their minds too much on their grief.

Ruby's caution was based on her own observation, but Polly had been a midwife for over 30 years and drew on her own experience of having a stillborn baby to support her suggestion that a self-help group may perpetuate the mother's grief.

Polly I had a stillbirth myself ... when I came here there was a group from SANDS and they came down. They were talking, there was a group talking to the midwives about what their group did. I found it very harrowing. Even after all those years, I found that harrowing because I thought to myself 'I wouldn't have liked that'. As I say, I thought to myself I wouldn't have liked it if that had been offered to me. Of course in those days there were no such things as support groups. But I wouldn't have liked it. I felt that it wasn't really healthy that they should be just making this a big thing in their life. What worries me is the effect on the mums. That's what worries me. Because I try to put myself ... I try to remember what it was like, and I wouldn't have liked it. They spoke about how they felt and how this happened and that happened and I felt it was as if they were grabbing on to this instead of trying to get over it. That was just how I felt. I really thought it was a bit unhealthy. I found it off-putting, I really did.

The possibility that self-help groups may be counterproductive to the extent that they may serve to prevent the grieving woman progressing through the stages of her grief is raised by McNeill-Taylor (1983) in the context of widowhood. Stroebe and Stroebe (1987) similarly discuss the risk that the woman may be hindered from moving beyond the 'widow' role.

Although this point was very real to the midwives who mentioned it, it is necessary to question its value. The members of the self-help group who appeared to be 'stuck' in their grief were only being observed in the group setting where self-disclosure is a feature and which may or may not have been typical of each woman's behaviour.

Additionally, it is impossible to assess whether group membership affected the duration of each woman's grief, because depth and duration of grief are highly individual. I would question whether the grief would have persisted anyway.

Group structure

That self-help groups are organised by lay people may serve to increase their sensitivity to the needs of their members, but difficulties may arise which may appear insoluble to people with little experience of group functioning (Murgatroyd & Woolfe, 1982). Tensions within the group may result in power struggles which reduce its effectiveness. On the other hand, if professionals are involved they may be used and allow themselves to be used inappropriately excessively. Assuming that the group is successful in resolving the concerns of the members, it may not know how to end itself in a constructive way, that is by passing on its knowledge to others who are at an earlier stage in the process.

The assumption of mutual experience

An assumption which underpins self-help is the significance of mutuality of experience, in that a person who has been through devastating grief, such as the loss of a baby, is better able to help and support another person going through it. The assumption that 'my grief is your grief' may deny the uniqueness of the other person's feelings and, perhaps, even trivialise them. This assumption is explicit in the work of Schiff, for bereaved parents (1977):

'What we had was something few could give them. We had experience. When they saw us, they saw the mother and father of a dead child, who were able to cope.'

The danger in this assumption was brought home to me when my father died and a well-meaning colleague wrote a condolence note telling me of her father's death two years earlier and how she knew what I was feeling. The differences between her background and mine were too vast for there to be any common ground and her presumptiousness further confused my already mixed feelings.

Leon (1990) recognises the uniqueness of grief when he warns us that the 'revival of individual conflicts during pregnancy and its loss' may limit the value of a group approach. I suggest that we recognise the assumption of commonality for what it is and handle it cautiously.

Evaluation

It is clear that, with only a few words of caution, midwives are generally happy to inform grieving mothers of the existence and role of perinatal bereavement support groups. We need to ask, though, to what extent midwives' confidence is justified. The need to evaluate the contribution of these groups is recognised by Tom-Johnson (1990) in her account, but research into their functioning is lacking.

An exception is found in the work of Lieberman (1979) who, with his colleagues, studied seven different self-help groups, including the Compassionate Friends, a group for bereaved parents (Davidson, 1979). Lieberman's data focus on bereaved parents' reasons for joining Compassionate Friends, rather than on the benefits of membership.

A researcher, who had earlier been associated with the work of Lieberman, found that involvement with Compassionate Friends served to protect the parents from the development of emotional problems (Videka-Sherman, 1982). She found that parents who had lost a child through death within the previous 18 months and were more active in the group were less likely to be depressed one year after the death than a similar group who contributed less to the organisation of the group and the support of other members. In interpreting these findings we must beware of assuming causality, as those parents who experienced their loss less severely, and perhaps were less depressed, may have been better able to help the other group members.

Researching the parents' experience of grief with the support of a self-help group would be highly sensitive, but evaluation research has been completed in other, similarly sensitive areas; examples include research on widows' grief and mourning (Raphael, 1984b), bereaved families (Williams & Polak, 1979), high-risk bereaved families (Parkes, 1980), women's consciousness-raising (Videka, 1979) and adjustment in the elderly (Lieberman & Gourash, 1979). The dilemmas and pitfalls of such sensitive, grief-related research are well-documented (Lieberman & Bond, 1979).

It appears that midwives are recommending self-help, as a way of helping grieving parents to adjust to their loss, without any research base. Inadequate knowledge of the functioning and benefits of self-help in this context, render the midwife vulnerable (Chalmers, 1993). It is, thus, imperative that we should undertake research into the effectiveness of this form of support; perhaps by seeking the views of those with good experiences of such a group and comparing their ideas with those whose experience was less successful.

Summary

While the presence of self-help groups is much valued by midwives and appears mainly beneficial, we must listen to the words of caution which come from a range of sources; these include the warning of Kalish (1985):

> 'This does not mean that participation in death-related self-help groups never leads to serious disturbance [but] such participation is extremely low risk and the potential rewards are substantial.'

Chapter 12
Future Childbearing

For reasons that I do not fully understand, the question of a future pregnancy invariably arises when health care providers think about perinatal loss. Although I never raised the topic, many of the midwives in my recent study (Mander, 1992d) thought that it was important to tell me about the prospect of the grieving mother embarking on another pregnancy. Some midwives illustrated how much our ideas have changed by disparagingly quoting 'traditional' advice:

Annie 'You can have another baby, you are young yet, it doesn't really matter.'

In quoting this comment, Annie was criticising the way it trivialises the mother's experience and denies the uniqueness of her lost baby; but it was presumably intended originally to reassure the mother and to persuade her to think positively about the future rather than dwell on the past. It may have, thus, been intended to 'cure', or at least curtail, the mother's grief. That this view still exists was impressed upon me by the relinquishing mothers I interviewed, many of whom were being or had been encouraged to consider the therapeutic value of another pregnancy.

Ursula's son was eight weeks old when we spoke and her anger and sorrow were still painfully obvious. This led her family to try to help:

Ursula Everybody round about keeps advising me to have another child to make me feel better. But I'm not going to have a child as a form of therapy.

Resuming sexual intercourse

Although the subsequent pregnancy has been the subject of much attention, the method of conception, sexual intercourse, has been largely neglected. The difficulty of re-establishing a loving, sexual relationship following perinatal death is apparent mainly from mothers' personal anecdotes.

Kohner and Henley (1992) show us how hard it may be for a couple

181

to enjoy even the human contact which may be quite independent of love-making. Physical comfort and support may be too much to ask of someone who feels they have nothing left to give. Even gentle warmth and cuddles demand a degree of relaxation which may be hard for a grieving parent.

Sexual intimacy following the death of a child was studied by Johnson (1984), showing that, while physical comfort may be appreciated, sexual intercourse is unlikely to be resumed until the couple are planning another pregnancy.

Differing patterns and rates of grieving may compound this difficulty because one partner is unable to respond to the other's tentative advances. Similarly, feelings of 'being ready for it', in terms of either grieving or simply inclination, may not coincide, escalating a cycle of tension and avoidance. Their resumption of sexual intercourse is likely to be delayed, as for any new parents, by the mother's traumatised genital area and lack of vaginal lubrication.

Hidden meanings exist in sexual intercourse for a couple who are grieving, such as memories of love-making, some months earlier, which began their baby's all-too-brief existence, recalling a more joyful and more carefree time (Borg & Lasker, 1982). The pleasurable nature of love-making may, thus, be regarded as inappropriate. Borg and Lasker describe the perilous downward spiral from 'I don't feel like it' to 'How could we?' to 'How could you think of it?'

The physical act of intercourse may serve as a further reminder of the birth and the death, as two mothers recounted (Kohner & Henley, 1992):

> 'She was the last person inside me and I didn't want to wipe out any part of that sacred memory.'
> 'Every time we make love I relive the birth.'

For either partner, fear of beginning another pregnancy which has the potential for further trauma may deter them from seeking the comfort of love-making. Many couples deeply regret the inability to give each other intimate, loving support when they most need it; but Borg and Lasker suggest that some may be relieved at the removal of anxieties about performance and conception which are inherent in sex.

Desiring to begin another pregnancy

The desire to begin another pregnancy may be interpreted differently. It may be a sign of recovery from the grief of perinatal loss, in the same way as remarriage may be a sign of adjustment to being widowed (Littlewood, 1992).

Johnson (1984) interprets his data in a similarly optimistic way, when he suggests that the wish for another pregnancy may be a growth-promoting affirmation of life. Unfortunately his data provide insufficient detail of either the depth of parental grief or the reasons for the hasty pregnancies for his conclusions to be accepted. Thus, this positive interpretation of rapid decision-making appears to be flawed.

Urgency and grieving

The more usual view of the urgent desire for another pregnancy as a relatively early stage of grieving is demonstrated in research by Giles (1970) and by Wolff *et al.* (1970). Giles interviewed 40 bereaved mothers in the early puerperium and shows their broad range of feelings about a future pregnancy. At one extreme, five mothers were doubtful of ever attempting another pregnancy, because their self-esteem was too low to allow them to contemplate success. At the opposite extreme was a similarly small group who were desperate to conceive again really quickly.

This group of desperate women probably equate with a similar, but larger group, in the study by Wolff *et al.* These researchers interviewed 50 bereaved mothers, also in the early postnatal period, but with a three-year follow-up, thus learning of both their plans as well as their pregnancies. An immediate pregnancy was planned by 40% of the mothers, but 50% actually conceived within three years. Wolff *et al.* (1970) regard these rapid pregnancies as examples of an immature response to the non-fulfillment of the women's fantasies of mother-hood.

Leon's psychotherapeutic approach (1990) interprets this reaction in terms of the mother's narcissism, self-esteem, or self-love. Clearly the mother's self-image has been irrevocably damaged by her perception of her failure to give birth to a healthy baby. Leon argues that for her, another, successful, pregnancy is the only route by which she may regain her equilibrium.

Deciding to begin another pregnancy

Making the decision about a future pregnancy may be influenced by a number of factors. Close family members as well as more casual acquaintances may urge the couple into parenthood (Borg & Lasker, 1982; Floyd, 1981). The woman's awareness of her own biological clock may hurry her decision. On the other hand, fears of a similar outcome may deter the couple from another attempt (Floyd, 1981).

The work of Wolff *et al.* shows us the large proportion, 50%, of bereaved mothers who decide that the chance is not worth taking, and for half of these the decision was made irrevocable by sterilisation.

Rowe *et al.* (1978) examined the association between having existing children and the decision to begin another pregnancy. This longitudinal study of 26 families grieving a perinatal death showed that those without living children were significantly more likely to embark on another pregnancy than those with children at home.

Timing

The timing of a future pregnancy is a source of concern; authors invariably consider the duration of the gap and often recommend a suitable time for the couple to plan a conception (Floyd, 1981). The recommended time varies, but six months to one year is usual (Kargar, 1990; Kohner & Henley, 1992; Klaus & Kennell, 1982b; Oglethorpe, 1989), but a flexible approach suggests waiting 'many months' (Kirk, 1984). Advising a woman to wait before beginning another pregnancy is emphasised as essential by Giles (1970), an obstetrician. He advocates that grieving mothers should wait for one year; his advice aggravated the upset felt by those mothers in his sample who were keen to conceive.

These exhortations are reminiscent of the experience of Rose (1990), a widowed psychotherapist who had listened to the advice and read the books and confidently expected her feelings to revert to normal one year after her bereavement. She convinced herself of the 12-month myth and that on the magical date her problems would end. She was shattered when she felt no better and eventually felt much worse on that date. Her experience warns us against being prescriptive about the duration of grief.

Rowe *et al.* (1978) illustrate the danger of such prescription when they went as far as to diagnose 'morbid grieving' when parents' grief lasted 12 to 20 months after perinatal bereavement. The need to avoid fixed time periods is endorsed by Lewis and Bourne (1989) who refute the implication that longer grief is automatically abnormal grief, suggesting that we should look at the person rather than the calendar before labelling grief 'abnormal'.

Reasons for waiting

The reasons for waiting to conceive are discussed by Kowalski (1987) and Oakley *et al.* (1984), who distinguish the physiological and the psychological factors, concluding that the mother's body is likely to be ready within three to six months, but her emotional state will need at least 12 months to recover.

Without recommending a time, Lewis and Page (1978) demonstrate the dangers of the mother becoming pregnant quickly after losing a baby and, hence, the importance of both the advice concerning waiting and the actual time gap. In a case study, a mother's inability to care for or relate to her healthy newborn daughter threatened the baby's survival. These psychotherapists attributed the mother's difficulty to her failure to mourn her stillborn first baby, who was born 12 months before his sister. By confronting the mother with her recollections of the first birth, the therapists forced her to begin the grieving which she had avoided, as evidenced by her second pregnancy. These authors regard a speedy pregnancy as avoiding the painfully difficult mourning of a perinatal death. Hence, the advice to wait.

Pregnancy and grieving

The effect of pregnancy on grieving derives from the incompatibility of these processes in one person. Pregnancy foreshortens grief, but the effect is temporary, holding the possibility that grief may re-emerge after the birth (Lewis & Bourne, 1989).

One of the reasons for the incompatibility of grief and pregnancy relates to the need in both for the mother to adopt a particular mental stance to complete her emotional task, as both involve sorting out inevitable ambivalent feelings (Lewis, 1979b). When grieving, she focuses on her sorrow at ending her relationship with the dead person by recalling and working through her memories of that person. When pregnant she optimistically begins to establish her new relationship with her child, largely by fantasising about this new person and how she will relate to them. This is part of the process known as 'bonding'.

As well as the essentially diametrically opposed emotional stances required, both processes are exclusive, to the extent that they both prevent other emotional work being effectively completed simultaneously.

Lewis and Bourne (1989) draw a picture of the mother's 'inner world' to explain this exclusivity; were it possible, this world would be inhabited by the dead baby she is grieving and the new baby she is starting to love. The internalisation of the images of the two babies simultaneously is prevented by the mother's fear that the new baby will be harmed by such close proximity to the dead baby. She, thus, blocks or unconsciously calls a halt to her grieving, which may. be resumed either when her anxieties about her unseen new baby are dealt with or possibly at some other unpredictable future time. Lewis (1979b) alerts us to the likelihood that this incomplete mourning may reappear in a pathological form, activated by unforeseen events.

It is apparent that a new pregnancy will deprive the mother of both time and space for grieving her lost baby (Bourne & Lewis, 1984). The long-term implications are difficult to foresee, but we may be certain that a mother who hurries or is hurried into another pregnancy is likely to find the experience unpleasant or even traumatic.

Conceiving and being pregnant

When the bereaved couple feel ready to embark on a pregnancy, their difficulties are far from over. In a retrospective epidemiological study, Vogel and Knox (1975) found that couples who had experienced perinatal or early infant death attempted to compensate their loss by a rapid pregnancy, resulting in a rise in the fertility rate of the sample in the year after bereavement. This increase was not maintained and the conception rate soon fell, to the extent that over a 5 year period there was a marked reduction in their fertility, alongside which, their success in childbearing was further reduced by a tendency for deaths to recur.

This observation of impaired childbearing following loss has also been noted in the context of parents who have lost a child through SIDS. The work of Mandell and Wolfe (1975) focused on subsequent pregnancies in 41 couples bereaved by SIDS. Of the mothers, 8 were keen to avoid pregnancy and used contraception. After one mother who was pregnant when bereaved gave birth prematurely, only 13 mothers had no problems with conceiving and carrying the pregnancy. Ten mothers experienced their first ever miscarriage, 2 of whom were subsequently infertile. Among this previously fertile group, the next pregnancy took between 15 months and 7 years to conceive. These 'problem pregnancy' rates are clearly higher than the expected infertility and miscarriage rates of 10% and 12% respectively.

On the basis of these data, Mandell and Wolfe propose that grieving is a psychological state which lowers the couple's childbearing ability. This suggestion is endorsed by the work of Vogel and Knox, which indicates that grieving couples' attempts to enlarge their families are frustrated by lower long-term fertility and associated with poorer outcomes. The effect of stress on fertility is well-established (Bancroft, 1989), but the effects of grief are less widely-known; these researchers suggest that grief may have a similarly adverse effect. Our care of grieving parents should include a warning that a, hopefully temporary, decline in their fertility may be expected.

Care in a subsequent pregnancy

In any future pregnancy it may be necessary to regard the mother as high-risk. This applies especially if the reasons for the death have not been identified, but it is necessary to consider whether the increased likelihood of a poor outcome (Vogel & Knox, 1975) puts this mother in need of particularly vigilant care (Fogel, 1981).

The demands on the woman who becomes pregnant after a perinatal loss are hugely increased; superimposed on all the physical and psychological tasks which pregnancy requires, she may not only have the demands of the additional investigations but she may also have the 'illness tasks' involved in adapting to the patient role (Clark & Affonso, 1976; Rubin, 1975; Parsons, 1951). Fogel (1981) discusses the subsequent pregnancy in terms of it being a crisis for the woman and her family.

Peplau (1976) lists four behaviours which help us to identify anxiety reaching the point of crisis in pregnancy:

(1) somatisation – when the woman draws attention to her distress through bodily signs
(2) acting out – physical activity or inactivity used to distract her attention from her distress
(3) introspection – withdrawal from the external world to focus on her inner conflict
(4) investigation – constant reading and questioning about her health status.

The demands of a crisis are added and crisis intervention may be appropriate to support her through this pregnancy. Support is offered in the following sequence (Fogel, 1981):

(1) the initial assessment of the mother and her problem
(2) deciding with her the appropriate interventions
(3) making the intervention
(4) anticipatory guidance to forestall any future crises.

If there are family members close by, the value of their input through the crisis should not be underestimated.

To avoid memories of sadness and loss, Kargar (1990) suggests that the mother's antenatal care should be provided 'well away from the hospital'. Whether such out-of-hospital care is consistent with the vigilant care which is required for this mother is questionable, but suitably intensive support may be more easily offered in a non-hospital setting.

The value of concentrated support, without high-tech interventions, during pregnancy has been shown to increase the rate of successful pregnancies in couples with a poor childbearing history (Stray-Pedersen & Stray-Pedersen, 1984). These researchers studied 195 couples who had had between 3 and 13 consecutive miscarriages. The couples were examined to exclude physical, hormonal or other causes for their recurrent miscarriages.

Of the 85 couples (43.6%) in whom no cause was identifiable, 61 subsequently conceived. Thirty-seven of these pregnant mothers were allocated to an experiment group for intensive 'tender loving care' during pregnancy and the remaining 24 served as controls and received routine antenatal care. The experiment group were given optimal psychological support, a weekly medical examination by one of the researchers and instructions to rest as much as possible and avoid heavy work and travelling. The control group were advised to avoid sex around the time of the previous miscarriages.

In the experiment group, 32 mothers (86%) gave birth to live, healthy, term babies whereas in the control group only 8 (33%) had a successful outcome. The authors claim that the difference is statistically highly significant.

While being concerned about the ethics of any women receiving care which is anything other than the best, this study shows the value of this form of low-tech intervention. Before deciding whether such care could or should be widely available we must consider its highly labour-intensive, and therefore costly, nature and also the possibility that the Hawthorne Effect may have been operating due to the close involvement of the researchers.

The value of more intensive antenatal care is endorsed by the recommendation that time should be made available for a bereaved mother to talk and ask questions about both the current pregnancy as well as the previous unsuccessful one (Lewis & Bourne, 1989; Sherr, 1989b). Contemplating support during pregnancy leads to the question of whether more intensive care in the form of counselling or psychotherapy has any advantages over the support already described. Oglethorpe (1989) states that analytical psychotherapy may be technically difficult at this time, has particular hazards and carries no marked benefits (Bourne, 1983; Bourne & Lewis, 1984; Apprey, 1987).

After the birth

The arrival of the new baby may resurrect in the mother many of the feelings associated with the loss of her previous baby:

Josie   In the case of the bereaved mother the baby is dead and it is all over, that is until she has a future pregnancy and all the memories will come flooding back.

If the mother's grieving is incomplete, she may suppress her strong feelings of loss which may continue to blank-out her emotions (Lewis, 1979b). The difficulty for the mother in establishing a relationship with a new baby while still grieving the loss of a previous one was shown by Caplan (1957). So, inevitably, her feelings of affection for her new baby may be diminished and her relationship with it impaired (Floyd, 1981; Klaus & Kennell, 1982b).

As discussed already, delayed grieving is a response which may be expected if a hasty pregnancy follows perinatal death (Bourne & Lewis,

1984; Lewis & Bourne, 1989; Lewis & Page, 1978; Lewis, 1979b; Sherr, 1989b).

The problems of an over-hasty conception are detailed in a case-study (Lewis & Page, 1978) in which a second child was born 12 months after her stillborn brother, making her an 'anniversary baby'. For anyone who has been bereaved, anniversaries are difficult (Kohner & Henley, 1992), but the conflict between celebrating a birth at the same time as recalling the 'death-day' engenders bewilderment in the parents (Bourne & Lewis, 1984; Lewis & Bourne, 1989).

Avoidance of an anniversary birth constitutes a further reason for delaying the next conception. It is necessary to be vigilant for these coincidences, either 'in prospect or in retrospect', in order to help the parents to open up and share any underlying feelings.

The replacement child syndrome

Although Oglethorpe (1989) defines a replacement child as either one who is specifically conceived to replace one who has died or a child forced by its family into this position, the term tends to be used rather loosely to describe any child who is born soon after a loss or disappointment (Floyd, 1981; Borg & Lasker, 1982; Bourne & Lewis, 1984; Lewis, 1979b).

In the seminal paper on this topic, Cain and Cain (1964) draw on their experience of six families who had suddenly lost a mature child through illness or accident. The severe psychiatric morbidity in, usually, the bereaved mother signified unresolved grief, which resulted in the albeit hesitant decision to replace the lost child. The authors describe the birth of a child into an environment totally bound up with the memory of the dead child. The parents were older, possibly in their 40s, and their expectation was hardly for an infant, as they were seeking a replacement for a mature child. The identification of the new child with its dead sibling was overpowering and constant comparisons were made. Unfortunately for the replacement child, quite unrealistic 'hyper-idealisation' of the dead sibling featured commonly.

In the context of relinquishment, Ursula, contemplating a 'replacement child', recognised the risk of 'idealising' the one who was relinquished, with the potential for trauma:

Ursula Another problem is that he is the perfect child. He has no bad points and will always be quite unique to me. Because when I first saw him he was perfect at his birth and every time I saw him after that he was being good. I s'pose that it's like meeting anybody for the first time, you don't get to know any of their bad points until you've met them a few times.

Cain and Cain focus on the prevalent psychiatric disturbances found among the replacement children, whose difficulties do not diminish as they grow older (Bourne & Lewis, 1984). Cain and Cain consider the family pathology engendered by well-meaning but ill-informed friends and professionals who had recommended 'having another'.

Whether this syndrome, derived from case studies following the deaths of older children, is applicable to perinatal loss merits consideration. Cain and Cain (1964) and Leon (1990) argue that the more limited investment in a fetus or neonate reduces the likelihood of such a severe reaction. Bluglass (1980), however, has demonstrated, in the context of SIDS, that problems of a similar nature do occur after the deaths of relatively young babies. Applying this knowledge to our practice, we must bear in mind that the risk of the replacement child syndrome increases when parents have no contact with or recollection of the dead baby (Leon, 1990).

Some elements of magical thinking may impinge upon this already complicated family situation (Lewis & Bourne, 1989), which may be linked by unconscious parental wishes to reincarnation fantasies. Bourne and Lewis (1984) tease out a connection between fantasies of the dead baby and the well-known phenomenon, mentioned already – anniversary birth.

The name of the dead child has only recently attracted concern, because it acknowledges the reality and the individuality of the child (Klaus & Kennell, 1982b). In thinking about any subsequent pregnancy the name assumes even greater significance; this is because the re-use of the same or a similar first name for a later child is considered indicative of pathological grief, that is, replacement child syndrome and may forewarn of attendant risks (Lewis, 1979b).

In their paper on this syndrome, Cain and Cain (1964) recount the confusion which the bereaved parents in their sample showed, by mistakenly addressing the replacement child by the name of the dead sibling. They suggest that this situation is aggravated by using a similar-sounding, perhaps gender-adjusted, name for the replacement child.

The underlying problem is spelt out by Bourne and Lewis (1984):

'We believe it something of a disaster for the next baby to be saddled with the name formerly intended for the one who died, adding to the danger that the new baby is only precariously differentiated from the dead one . . .'

These authors go on to suggest that we, as health care providers, are ideally situated to prevent names being re-used in this way.

These researchers are suitably wary of the damage experienced by a 'replacement child' and regard the name as an important indicator. Unfortunately they regard the name as little more than a label or perhaps a diagnostic tool. The true significance of the name is discussed by Raphael-Leff (1991) in terms of it being a 'live myth' which is bestowed upon the child. She regards the name as an attribution, rather than a mere label. It represents the parents' hopes and aspirations for their child. Although the name may appear to represent just a character in a soap opera or a pop singer, to the parents this may be the pinnacle of achievement, their ultimate hopes for their child.

Raphael-Leff traces the use of different names according to the prevailing cultural and religious beliefs. The practice in the UK of using the same first name through the generations is becoming uncommon, though this certainly applied in my own family where my father and two brothers all used the same name!

Thus, the name may be seen to represent desirable qualities with which the parents hope that the child will be blessed. This leads us to question whether it is really inappropriate to re-use a name because the person for whom it was intended has died. Connolly (1989b) reports the practice in the west of Ireland of giving the same name to a sibling of a dead child. He maintains that this is acceptable because of what the name represents, regardless of whether it has been used previously.

Summary

It is clear that embarking on another pregnancy after perinatal loss carries a range of hazards. For the mother, the pregnancy itself may be evidence of inadequate grieving, with the likelihood of that grieving being resurrected at some unpredictable future time. For the child, the chances of, first, being conceived and, second, of surviving the perinatal period are reduced. In the event of replacement child syndrome, the risk of psychological trauma to the child/person is immeasurable.

However, the original reason for the conception of the child who was lost is not affected by the loss of that child. The need for a child, for whatever reason, still pertains within the family; so the next child, if there is one, should not necessarily be regarded as a replacement, but as a wanted child.

Research evidence suggests that, if necessary, appropriate interventions are available to help the mother to achieve success in both childbearing and psychological terms.

Thus, our concerns for the welfare of the family and a subsequent child may not always be justified and in the event of inappropriate grief responses our interventions to help the family are able to prevent morbidity.

Conclusion
Benefits and Meanings

To conclude, I draw out two interrelated themes which have emerged through this book. Although we tend to think automatically of the tragic nature of perinatal loss, there may be positive aspects. An example is the loving relationship which is the precursor to grief, which I focused on in the early chapters; included with this should be the personal growth and development which follows grief.

Findings of personal growth through increased self-knowledge emerged from a recent study of mothers' experiences of miscarriage (Bansen & Stevens, 1992), together with heightened perceptions of both the joys and trauma of life, which were associated with an increased sense of responsibility. This manifested itself in the mother assuming more control over her life and health.

These positive aspects are similar to those found in a study of parental relationships after the death of a child (Klass, 1986). An increased awareness of their priorities and recognition of their own strength was associated with a new sensitivity to the feelings and the pain of others.

Helmrath and Steinitz (1978) identified benefits in terms of improved communication between bereaved parents. Those who were able to share their feelings increased their mutual trust and felt that this was essential to the resolution of their grief. The couples also thought that the quality of their relationship had improved and perceived the loss of their baby as an opportunity for growth.

As the experience of loss generally has provided a stimulus for major creative efforts, so too has the experience of perinatal loss. Borg and Lasker (1982) list women, such as Mary Shelley, Anais Nin and Harriet Beecher Stowe, who were thus inspired. Benoliel (1985) shows how childhood grief later found artistic expression in the work of Edvard Munch and Kathe Kollwitz.

The extent to which these positive aspects affect the feelings of loss depends on the unique meaning which the mother attaches to her experience. The meaning which the pregnancy holds for her influences her grief; the meaning is highly individual and may include elements ranging from narcissism to a search for adulthood (Raphael-Leff, 1991).

Leon (1992) alerts us to the dangers of regarding perinatal loss as 'solely the loss of a baby'; warning us that at least three separate dimensions of loss must be considered – individual, marital and family losses.

The meaninglessness of the loss and, possibly, of life itself features in the later stages of acute grief (Parkes, 1976). The mother's interpretation of her loss determines the extent to which she feels able to make sense of her situation; which, in turn, determines our care. As carers we are able to help her find the meaning of her loss; an example is how we provide opportunities and allow her space to fathom the unique meaning of her loss. The family is similarly better able to cope if it is able to find meaning (Cook & Oltjenbruns, 1989).

As is so often the case, we are able to learn from the example of children, in whom the dynamic process by which the meaning of loss develops as the child sibling matures is clearly apparent. This is partly due to the child's open and uninhibited search for meaning, whereas in adults that search is more secretive.

In the same way as the meaning of her pregnancy determines her grief if the pregnancy is lost, so too the meaning the mother attributes to her child influences her response if her child has a handicap.

While her reaction to her loss is influenced by a wide range of unknown factors, including the meaning and significance of her loss, so too is her behaviour. The mother's response is affected by personal and cultural experiences which we may not share and which, to us, make her behaviour incomprehensible, yet to her these behaviours and rituals are imbued with profound significance, deserving respect.

We are warned to avoid assumptions, especially of the meaning of the pregnancy and its loss (Worden, 1992). While we may be safer assuming that her loss constitutes an incapacitating tragedy, we should be prepared for and accepting of other reactions. The assumptions of some, such as the gurus who trivialise miscarriage with accusations of it being 'magnified into a catastrophe' (Bourne & Lewis, 1991), serve only to reinforce Worden's warning.

As I have suggested already, the benefits of loss and grief are not immediately obvious. The ideas of Marris (1986) provide a helpful framework which illuminate the enduring benefits of the all too familiar pain. Marris believes that we create 'structures of meaning', which comprise an organised set of perceptions and beliefs which help us to make sense of our experiences in relation to the context in which they happen. Our structures of meaning preserve an element of continuity, by providing a system through which we are able to integrate new experiences into an existing mental framework. This is clearly essential when continuity is as fundamentally threatened as it is during bereavement.

Marris' hypothesis suggests that grief constitutes a reaction to the disintegration of the structure of meaning associated with the lost relationship. Thus, grief comprises efforts to transform the meaning of the relationship to allow continuity to be restored.

For these reasons, some degree of discomfort or distress is an inevitable consequence of loss. It needs to be perceived as a constructive, rather than just an inevitable, experience which helps us to adapt to maintain the continuity of life as shown in the examples given by Craig (1977).

In this book I began by looking at the meanings of the words commonly used when thinking about loss. I close by drawing together the recurring themes of the meaning of the loss itself and the long-term and intrinsic benefits of grief.

References

Aamodt, A.M. (1982) Examining Ethnography for Nurse Researchers. *Western Journal of Nursing Research*, **4**(2), 209–21.

Adams, M. & Prince, J. (1990) Care of the Grieving Parent with Special Reference to Stillbirth. In: Alexander, J., Levy, V. & Roch, S. *Post Natal Care: A Research-based Approach*. Macmillan Education, London.

Adams, R. (1990) *Self-help, Social Work and Empowerment*, Macmillan Education, Basingstoke.

Adshead, G. & Dickenson, D. (1993) Why Do Doctors and Nurses Disagree? In: Dickenson, D. & Johnson, M. *Death, Dying and Bereavement*. Open University and Sage, London.

Aggleton, P. & Homans, H. (1988) *Social Aspects of AIDS*. Falmer Press Ltd., London.

Allingham, M. (1952) *Tiger in the Smoke*. Chatto & Windus, London.

Almond, B. (1990) Personal issues and personal dilemmas. In: chapter 12, (ed. B. Almond). *AIDS, a moral issue: The ethical, legal and social aspects*, Macmillan Press Ltd., Basingstoke.

Anon (1990) We all know better: the feelings. *The Guardian*, 29 November, p. 21.

Anon (1991) Editorial Bereavement – Who Counsels the Counsellor? *Journal of Nurse-Midwifery*, **36**(3), 151–2.

Anon (1993a) A cry for help. *Nursing Times*, **89**(4), 29–30.

Anon (1993b) A Student's Story. In: Dickenson, D. & Johnson, M. *Death, Dying and Bereavement*. Open University and Sage, London.

Apprey, M. (1987) Projective identification and maternal misconception in disturbed mothers. *British Journal of Psychotherapy*, **4**, 5–22.

Aradine, C.R. & Ferketich, S. (1990) The Psychological Impact of Premature Birth on Mothers and Fathers. *Journal of Reproductive and Infant Psychology*, **8**(2), 75–86.

Atkinson, F.I. (1991) Survey Design and Sampling. In: *The Research Process in Nursing*, (ed. D.F.S. Cormack), 2nd edn. Blackwell Scientific Publications, Oxford.

Awoonor-Renner, S. (1993) I Desperately Needed to See my Son. In: Dickenson, D. & Johnson, M. *Death, Dying and Bereavement*. Open University and Sage, London.

Baggaley, S. (1993) Personal Communication.

Bailey, R. & Clarke, M. (1991) *Stress and Coping in Nursing*. Chapman & Hall Ltd., London.

Bancroft, J.H.J. (1989) *Human Sexuality and Its Problems*. Churchill Livingstone, Edinburgh.

Bannister, D. & Fransella, F. (1986) *Inquiring man: The psychology of personal constructs*, 3rd edn. Croom Helm Ltd., London.

Bansen, S.S. & Stevens, H.A. (1992) Women's experience of miscarriage in early pregnancy. *Journal of Nurse-Midwifery*, **37**(2), 84–90.

Barker, J. (1983) *Volunteer Bereavement Counselling Schemes*. Age Concern Research Unit, London.

Barlow, J. (1992) Social Issues: An Overview. In Bury, J., Morrison, V. & McLachlan, S. *Working With Women and AIDS: Medical, Social and Counselling Issues*. Tavistock/Routledge, London.

Beard, P. (1989) A Bereaved Child. *Nursing Times*, **85**(11), 59–61.

Becker, P.T., Grunwald, P.C., Moorman, J. & Stuhr, S. (1991) Outcomes of Developmentally Supportive Nursing Care for VLBW Infants. *Nursing Research*, **40**(3), 150–55.

Bender, H. (1981) Experiences in Running a Staff Group. *Journal of Child Psychotherapy*, **7**, 152–9.

Bender, H. & Swan-Parente, A. (1983) Pscychological and Psychotherapeutic Support of Staff and Parents in an Intensive Care Baby Unit. In: Davis, J.A., Richards, M.P.M. & Roberton, N.R.C. *Parent–Baby Attachment in Premature Infants*. Croom Helm Ltd., London.

Benfield, D.G., Leib, S.A. & Reuter, J. (1976) Grief Responses of parents after referral of the critically ill newborn to a regional center. *New England Journal of Medicine*, **294**, 975–8.

Benjamin, M. (1993) The First Day. In: Dickenson, D. & Johnson, M. *Death, Dying and Bereavement*. Open University and Sage, London.

Benoliel, J.Q. (1985) Loss and Adaptation: Circumstances, Contingencies and Consequences. *Death Studies*, **9**, 217–33.

Beszterczey, A. (1977) Staff Stress in a Newly-developed Palliative Care Service. *Canadian Psychiatric Association Journal*, **22**, 347–53.

Bluglass, K. (1980) Psychiatric Morbidity After Cot Death, *The Practitioner*, **224**, 533–9.

Blumberg, B. Golbus, M.S. & Hansen, K.H. (1975) The Psychological Sequelae of Abortion Performed for a Genetic Indication. *American Journal of Obstetrics and Gynecology*, **122**, 799–808.

Bond, M. (1986) *Stress and Self-awareness: A Guide for Nurses*. Heinemann Ltd., London.

Bond, S. & Rhodes, T.Y. (1990) HIV Infection and Community Midwives: Knowledge and Attitudes. *Midwifery*, **6**(2), 86–92.

Bond, S., Rhodes, T., Philips, P. & Tierney, A. (1990) Knowledge and Attitudes. *Nursing Times*, **86**(45), 49–51.

Bor, R. (1990) The Family and HIV/AIDS. *AIDS Care*, **2**(4), 409–12.

Bor, R. (1991) The ABC of AIDS Counselling. *Nursing Times*, **87**(1), 32–5.

Borg, S. & Lasker, J. (1982) *When Pregnancy Fails*. Routledge/Kegan Paul International Ltd., London.

Bouchier, P., Lambert, L. & Triseliotis, J. (1991) *Parting with a child for adoption: the mother's perspective*. British Agencies for Adoption and Fostering Discussion Series; 14, London.

Bourne, S. (1968) The Psychological Effects of Stillbirth on Women and Their

Doctors. *Journal of Royal College of General Practitioners,* **16**, 103–12.

Bourne, S. (1979) Coping with Perinatal Death. *Midwife, Health Visitor & Community Nurse,* Feb, pp. 59 and 62.

Bourne, S. & Lewis, E. (1984) Pregnancy After Stillbirth or Neonatal Death. *Lancet,* 8393 (ii), 31–3.

Bourne, S. & Lewis, E. (1991) Perinatal Bereavement: A Milestone and Some New Dangers. *British Medical Journal,* **302**, 1167–8.

Bowlby, J. (1958) The Nature of the Child's Tie to His Mother. *International Journal of Psychoanalysis,* **30**, 350.

Bowlby, J. (1961) Processes of Mourning. *International Journal of Psychoanalysis,* **44**, 317.

Bowlby, J. (1969) *Attachment and Loss Volume 1: Attachment.* The Hogarth Press, London.

Bowlby, J. (1977) The Making and Breaking of Affectional Bonds I & II. *British Journal of Psychiatry,* **130**, 201–10 and 421–31.

Bowlby, J. (1980) *Attachment and Loss Volume III: Loss, Sadness and Depression.* The Hogarth Press, London.

Boxall, J. & Whitby, C. (1983) The Role of the Nurse in Mother–Baby Interaction. In: Davis, J.A., Richards, M.P.M. & Roberton, N.R.C. *Parent–Baby Attachment in Premature Infants,* Croom Helm Ltd., London.

Brand, H.J. (1989) The Influence of Sex Differences on the Acceptance of Infertility. *Journal of Reproductive and Infant Psychology,* **7**(2), 129–31.

Brazelton, T.B. (1973) *Neonatal Behavioural Assessment Scale.* Spastic International Medical Publications, London.

Breen, D. (1978) The Mother and the Hospital. In: *Tearing the Veil: Essays of Feminity,* (ed. S. Lipshitz), Routledge/Kegan Paul International Ltd., London.

Bretherton, I. (1987) New Perspectives on Attachment Relations. In *Handbook of Infant Development,* (ed. J.D. Osofsky), Wiley, New York.

Brettle, R.P. & Leen, C.L.S. (1991) The Natural History of HIV & AIDS in Women. *AIDS,* **5**(11), 1283–92.

Brierley, J. (1988) Management of Perinatal Death. *Midwife Health Visitor & Community Nurse,* **24**(3), 80–4.

Brooks, T. (1989) *Best of Health.* Andersen Consulting, *Sunday Times,* London.

Brown, Y. (1992) The Crisis of Pregnancy Loss: A Team Approach to Support. *Birth,* **19**(2), 82–9.

Brown, M.A. & Powell-Cope, G.M. (1991) AIDS Family Caregiving: Transitions Through Uncertainty. *Nursing Research,* **40**(8), 338–44.

Bryan, E. (1992) Twins and Higher Multiple Births: A Guide to Their Nature and Nurture. Arnold (Edward) (Publishers) Ltd., Sevenoaks, Kent.

Buckman, R. (1993) Breaking Bad News: Why is it still so difficult? In: Dickenson, D. & Johnson, M. *Death, Dying and Bereavement.* Open University and Sage, London.

Burnard, P. & Morrison, P. (1991) Client-centred Counselling: A study of nurses' attitudes. *Nurse Education Today,* **11**(2), 104–9.

Bury, J. (1992) *Women's Issues.* Conference Paper at 3rd European Conference for Nurses in AIDS Care, October, Edinburgh.

Cain, A.C. & Cain, B.S. (1964) On Replacing a Child. *Journal of the American Academy of Child Psychiatry*, **3**, 433–56.

Cain, A.C., Erickson, M.E., Fast, I. & Vaughan, R. (1964) Children's Disturbed Reaction to their Mother's Miscarriage. *Psychosomatic Medicine*, **26**, 58–66.

Callan, V.J. & Hennessy, J.F. (1989) Psychological Adjustment to Infertility: A Unique Comparison of Two Groups of Infertile Women, Mothers and Women Childless by Choice. *Journal of Reproductive and Infant Psychology*, **7**(2), 105–12.

Cameron, J. & Parkes, C.M. (1983) Terminal Care: Evaluation of Effects on Surviving Family of Care Before and After Bereavement. *Postgraduate Medical Journal*, **59**, 73–8.

Campbell, A.V. (1979) The Meaning of Death and Ministry to the Dying. In *Terminal Care*, (ed. D. Doyle), Churchill Livingstone, Edinburgh.

Campbell, E. (1985) *The Childless Marriage: An Exploratory Study of Couples Who Do Not Want Children*. Tavistock Publications Ltd., London.

Caplan, A.L., Blank, R.H. & Merrick, J.C. (1992) *Compelled Compassion: Government Intervention in the Treatment of Critically Ill Newborns*. Humana Press, Totowa, New Jersey.

Caplan, G. (1957) Psychological aspects of maternity care. *American Journal of Public Health*, **47**, 25.

Caplan, G. (1961) *An Approach to Community Mental Health*. Tavistock Publications Ltd., London.

Carovano, K. (1991) More Than Mothers and Whores: Redefining the AIDS Prevention Needs of Women. *International Journal of Health Services*, **21**(1), 131–42.

Carter, D. (1991) Quantitative Research. In: Cormack, D. *The Research Process in Nursing*, 2nd edn, Blackwell Scientific Publications, Oxford.

Catania, J.A., Turner, H.A., Choi, K.H. & Coates, T.J. (1992) Coping with death anxiety: help-seeking and social support among gay men with various HIV diagnoses. *AIDS*, **6**, 999–1005.

Cathcart, F. (1989) Coping with Distress. *Nursing Times*, **85**(42), 33–5.

Chalmers, I. (1993) Effective Care in Midwifery: Research, the Profession and the Public. *Midwives Chronicle*, **106**(1260), 3–13.

Chambers (1981) *Chambers Twentieth Century Dictionary*, (ed. A.M. Macdonald), Chambers (W. & R.) Ltd., Edinburgh.

Chaney, P.S. (1981) *Dealing with Death and Dying: Nursing Skillbook*. Intermed Communications Ltd., Horsham, Pennsylvania.

Chevenert, M. (1978) *Special Techniques in Assertiveness Training for Women in Health Professions*. Mosby, St Louis.

Chitty, G.S., *et al.* (1991) Effectiveness of Routine Ultrasonography in Detecting Fetal Structural Abnormalities in a Low-risk Population. *British Medical Journal*, **303** (68111), 1165–9.

Chrystie, I.L., Palmer, S.J., Kenney, A. & Banatvala, J.E. (1992) HIV seroprevalence among women attending antenatal clinics in London. *Lancet*, 8789 (**339**), 364.

Clark, A.L. & Affonso, D. (eds) (1976) *Childbearing: A Nursing Perspective*. F.A. Davis & Co., Philadelphia.

Clark, G.T. (1991) To the Edge of Existence: Living Through Grief. *Phenomenology and Pedagogy*, Fall Issue.

Cole, A. (1993) Vital Support. *Nursing Times*, **89**(13), 16–17.

Collins, M. (1986) Care for Families Following Stillbirth and First Week Deaths, *Midwives Chronicle*, **99**(1176), January Suppl., xiii–xv.

Connolly, K.D. (1989a) Factors Affecting Grief Following Pregnancy Loss. In: van Hall, E.V. & Everaerd, W. *The Free Woman: Women's Health in the 1990s*. Parthenon, Carnforth.

Connolly, K.D. (1989b) *Factors Affecting Grief Following Pregnancy Loss.* 9th International Congress of Psychosomatic Obstetrics and Gynaecology, Amsterdam.

Cook, A.S. & Dworkin, D.S. (1992) *Helping the Bereaved: Therapeutic Interventions for Children, Adolescents and Adults.* Basic Books, USA.

Cooper, J.D. (1980) Parental Reactions to Stillbirth. *British Journal of Social Work*, **10**, 55–69.

Craig, Y. (1977) The Bereavement of Parents and their Search for Meaning. *British Journal of Social Work*, **7**(1) 41–54.

Crawley, P. (1983) 'Angels in Hell' Interview by A. Shearer. *The Guardian*, 29 June.

Critchley, L. (1992) Women and AIDS: Why Ignorance is Far from Bliss. *The Guardian*, 21 May.

Cullberg, J. (1971) Mental Reactions of Women to Perinatal Death. In: *Proceedings of the Third Congress of Psychosomatic Medicine in Obstetrics and Gynaecology, Basel*, Karger, Switzerland.

Cunningham, C.C., Morgan, P.A. & McGucken, R.B. (1984) Down's Syndrome: Is dissatisfaction with disclosure of diagnosis inevitable? *Developmental Medicine & Child Neurology*, **26**, 33–9.

de Chateau, P. (1980) Neonatal Capacity for Early Interaction and Its Long-term Consequences. In: Prill, H.-J. & Stauber, M. *Advances in Psychosomatic Obstetrics and Gynaecology*. Springer-Verlag, Berlin.

de Graaf, R., Van Wesenbeeck, I. & van Zessen, G. (1993) The Effectiveness of Condom Use in Hetereosexual Prostitution in the Netherlands. *AIDS*, **7**(2), 265–9.

de Leeuw, R. (1989) Coping with Neonatal Death in a NICU. In: van Hall, E.V. & Evaraerd, W. *The Free Woman: Women's Health in the 1990s*. Parthenon, Carnforth.

Darbyshire, P. (1992) Telling Stories, Telling Moments. *Nursing Times*. **88**(1), 22–4.

Davidson, G. (1977) Death of the Wished-for Child: A case study. *Death Education*, **1**, 265.

Davidson, H. (1979) Development of a Bereaved Parents Group. In: Lieberman, M.A., Borman, L.D. *et al. Self-help Groups for Coping With Crisis.* Jossey Bass, San Francisco.

Davis, D.L., Stewart, M. & Harmon, R.J. (1988) Perinatal Loss: Providing Emotional Support for Bereaved Parents. *Birth*, **15**(4) 242–6.

Davis, J.A. (1983) Ethical Issues in Neonatal Intensive Care. In: Davis, J.A., Richards, M.P.M. & Roberton, N.R.C. *Parent–Baby Attachment in Premature Infants.* Croom Helm Ltd., London.

Denenberg, R. (1992) Pregnant Women and HIV in ACT UP/New York

Women and AIDS Book Group. *Women, AIDS and Activism.* South End Press, Boston.

Denzin, N. (1970) *The Research Act in Sociology: A Theoretical Introduction to Sociological Methods.* Butterworth & Co. Ltd., London.

DOH (1991) *Report of Confidential Enquiries into Maternal Deaths in the United Kingdom 1985–7.* HMSO, London.

Dick, S. (1992) Positive Support. *Nursing Times,* **88**(44), 46–8.

Diekelmann, N. (1992) Show Some Emotion. *Nursing Times,* **88**(27), 39.

Donnai, P., Charles, N. & Harris, R. (1981) Attitudes of Patients to 'Genetic' Termination of Pregnancy. *British Medical Journal,* **282** 621–2.

Dor, J. et al. (1977) An Evaluation of the Etiologic Factors in Therapy in 665 Infertile Couples. *Fertility and Sterility,* **28**(7), 718–22.

Douglas, J. (1992) Black Women's Health Matters: Putting Black Women on the Research Agenda. In: Roberts, H. *Women's Health Matters,* p 33. Routledge, London.

Drever, J. (1964) *A Dictionary of Psychology.* Penguin, London.

Druery, K. (1992) Bereavement Support in a Maternity Unit. *Midwives Information and Resource Service Midwifery Digest,* **2**(2), 223–5.

Dunlop, R.J. & Hockley, J.M. (1990) *Terminal Care Support Teams.* Oxford University Press.

Dunn, D.T., Newell, M.L., Ades, A.E. & Peckham, C.S. (1992) Risk of HIV infection through breastfeeding. *Lancet,* **340**(8819), 585–9.

Dunn, J.B. (1975) Consistency and Change in Styles of Mothering. In: *Parent–Infant Interaction,* CIBA Foundation Symposium 33, Elsevier Science Publishers, Amsterdam.

Durham, T.W., McCammon, S.L., Allison, E.J. (1985) The Psychological Impact of Disaster on Rescue Personnel. *Annals of Emergency Medicine,* **14**(7), 664–8.

Dyer, M. (1992) Stillborn – Still Precious. *Midwives Information and Resource Service Midwifery Digest,* **2**(2), 341–4.

Dyregrov, A. (1991) *Grief in Children: A Handbook for Adults.* Kingsley (Jessica) Publishers, London.

Dyregrov, A. & Matthieson, S.B. (1987) Similarities and Differences in Mothers' and Fathers' Grief Following the Death of an Infant. *Scandinavian Journal of Psychology,* **28**, 1–15.

Dyregrov, A. (1988) The Loss of a Child: The Sibling's Perspective. In: *Motherhood and Mental Illness 2: Causes and Consequences,* (eds R. Kumar & N. Brockington). Wright, London.

Elizur, E. & Kauffman, M. (1983) Factors Influencing the Severity of Childhood Bereavement Reactions. *American Journal of Orthopsychiatry,* **53**, 668–76.

Ellison, G. (1990) Through the Darkest Hour. *Community Outlook,* November, pp 4–6.

Engel, G.C. (1961) Is Grief a Disease? A Challenge for Medical Research. *Psychosomatic Medicine,* **23**, 18–22.

Epstein, J. (1989) Organising a Bereavement Counselling Service. In: *Death, Dying and Bereavement,* (ed. L. Sherr). Blackwell Scientific Publications, Oxford.

European Collaborative Study (1991) Children born to women with HIV infection: Natural history and risk of transmission. *Lancet,* **337**(8736), 253–60.

Fairbairn, G. (1992) When a Baby Dies – A Father's View. In: Dickenson, D. & Johnson, M. *Death, Dying and Bereavement.* Open University and Sage, London.

Farrant, W. (1985) Who's for Amniocentesis? The Politics of Prenatal Screening. In: *The Sexual Politics of Reproduction,* (ed. H. Homans), chapter 7. Gower Publishing Co. Ltd., Aldershot.

Field, P.A. & Morse, J.M. (1987) *Nursing Research: The Application of Qualitative Approaches.* Croom Helm Ltd., London.

Fielding, N.G. & Lee, R.M. (1991) *Using Computers in Qualitative Research.* Sage Publications Ltd., London.

Firth, S. (1993) Cross-cultural Perspectives on Bereavement. In: Dickenson, D. & Johnson, M. *Death, Dying and Bereavement.* Open University and Sage, London.

Fitzpatrick, R., Boulton, M. & Hart, G. (1989) Gay men's sexual behaviour in response to AIDS. In: *Social Representations, Social Practices,* (eds P. Aggleton, G. Hart & P. Davies). Falmer Press Ltd., London.

Floyd, C.C. (1981) Pregnancy After Reproductive Failure. *American Journal of Nursing,* **81,** 2050–3.

Fogel, C.I. (1981) High Risk Pregnancy. In: Fogel, C.I. & Woods, N.F. *Health Care of Women: A Nursing Perspective.* Mosby, St Louis.

Forrest, G. (1989) Care of the Bereaved After Perinatal Death. In: Chalmers, I., Enkin, M. & Keirse, M.J.N.C. *Effective Care in Pregnancy and Childbirth,* **2.** Oxford University Press.

Forrest, G.C. (1983) Mourning Perinatal Death. In: Davis, J.A., Richards, M.P.M. & Roberton, N.R.C. *Parent–Baby Attachment in Premature Infants.* Croom Helm Ltd., London.

Forrest, G.C., Standish, E. & Baum, J.D. (1982) Support after perinatal death: a study of support and counselling after perinatal bereavement. *British Medical Journal,* **285,** 1475–9.

Foster, D.J., O'Malley, J.E. & Koocher, G.P. (1981) The Parent Interviews. In: *The Damocles Syndrome: Psychosocial Consequences of Surviving Childhood Cancer,* (eds J.E. O'Malley & G.P. Koocher). McGraw Hill, New York.

Frank, D.I. (1984) Counselling the Infertile Couple, *Journal of Psychosocial Nursing,* **22**(5), 17–23.

Freilich, M. (1979) Fieldwork: An Introduction. In: Freilich, M. *Marginal Natives: Anthropologists at Work.* Harper & Row, New York.

Friedman, T. (1989) Infertility and Assisted Reproduction. In: *Psychological Aspects of Obstetrics and Gynaecology* (ed. M.R. Oates). Baillière Tindall, London.

Friedman, T. & Gath, D. (1989) The Psychiatric Consequences of Spontaneous Abortion. *British Journal of Psychiatry,* **155,** 810–3.

Friend, B. (1992) Invisible Women. *Nursing Times,* **88**(49), 18.

Freud, S. (1917/59) Mourning and Melancholia. *Collected Papers.* Basic Books, New York. (Originally published in 1917.)

Fulton, R. & Gottesman, D.J. (1980) Anticipatory Grief: A Psychosocial Concept Reconsidered. *British Journal of Psychiatry,* **137,** 45–54.

Gans, H.J. (1982) The Participant Observer as a Human Being: Observations on the Personal Aspects of Fieldwork. In: Burgess, R.G. *Field Research: A Sourcebook and Field Manual*. Allen & Unwin (Publishers) Ltd., London.

Garber, J. & Seligman, M.E.P. (1980) *Human Helplessness: Theory and Applications*. Academic Press, New York.

Gartner, A. & Reissman, F. (1984) *The Self-help Revolution*, Human Sciences Press, New York.

Gayton, T. (1991) Life after Death, *The Guardian*, 27 February.

George, R.J.D. (1992) Coping with death anxiety – trying to make sense of it all. *AIDS*, **6**, 1037–8.

Gerber, I., Weiner, A., Battin, D. & Arkin, A. (1975) Grief Therapy to the Aged Bereave. In: *Bereavement: its Psychological Aspects*, (eds B. Schoenberg & I. Gerber). Columbia UP, New York.

Gibb, D.M.L. & Newell, M.L. (1992) HIV Infection in Children. *Archives of Disease in Childhood*, **67**, 138–41.

Giles, P.F.H. (1970) Reactions of Women to Perinatal Death. *Australian and New Zealand Journal of Obstetrics and Gynaecology*, **10**, 207–10.

Glaser, B.G. & Strauss, A.L. (1965) *Awareness of Dying*. Aldine Publishing, Chicago.

Goedert, J.J., Duliege, A.-M., Amos, C.I., Felton, S. & Biggar, R.J. (1991) High risk of HIV infection for first born twins. *Lancet*, **338**(8781), 1471–4.

Gohlish, M.C. (1985) Stillbirth, *Midwife Health Visitor and Community Nurse*, **21**(1), 16.

Gorer, G. (1965) *Death, Grief and Mourning in Contemporary Britain*, Cresset Press, London.

Grace, J.T. (1989) Development of Maternal–Fetal Attachment During Pregnancy. *Nursing Research*, **38**(4), 228–32.

Green, J.M., Statham, H. & Snowdon, C. (1993) Women's Knowledge of Prenatal Screening Tests. *Journal of Reproductive and Infant Psychology*, **11**(1), 31–40.

Grossman, K., Thane, K. & Grossman, K.E. (1981) Maternal Tactual Contact of the Newborn After Various Postpartum Conditions of Mother–Infant Contact. *Developmental Psychology*, **17**(1), 58–69.

Grubb, C.A. (1976) Body Image Concerns of a Multipara in the Situation of Intrauterine Fetal Death. *Maternal Child Nursing*, **5**, 93.

Guillemin, J.H. & Holmstrom, L.L. (1986) *Mixed Blessings: Intensive Care for Newborns*. Oxford University Press.

Handsfield, H.H. (1988) Editorial. *Journal of American Medical Association*, **260**(13), 1943–4.

Hardgrove, C. & Warrick, L.H. (1974) How Shall We tell the Children? *American Journal of Nursing*, **74**(3), 448–50.

Harlow, H.F. & Harlow, M.K. (1966) Learning to Love. *American Scientist*, **54**, 244–72.

Harmon, R.J., Glicken, A.D. & Siegel, R.E. (1984) Neonatal Loss in the Intensive Care Nursery: Effects on Maternal Grieving and Program for Intervention. *Journal of the American Academy of Child Psychiatry*, **23**, 68–71.

Harris, B.G. (1986) Induced Abortion. In: Rando, T. *Parental Loss of a Child*, Research Press, Champaign, Illinois.

Harris, M. (1968) *The Rise of Anthropological Theory.* Thomas Y. Crowell, New York.

Heller, T. (1993) Personal and Medical Memories from Hillsborough. In: Dickenson, D. & Johnson, M. *Death, Dying and Bereavement.* Open University and Sage, London.

Helmrath, T.A. & Steinitz, E.M. (1978) Death of an Infant: Parental Grieving and the Failure of Social Support. In: Rando, T.A. *Parental Loss of a Child.* Research Press, Champaign, Illinois.

Hepburn, M. (1992) Pregnancy and HIV: Screening, Counselling and Services. In: Bury, J., Morrison, V. & McLachlan, S. *Working with Women and AIDS: Medical, Social and Counselling Issues.* Tavistock/Routledge, London.

Herbert, M. & Sluckin, A. (1985) A Realistic Look at Mother–Infant Bonding. In: *Recent Advances in Perinatal Medicine: 2,* (ed. M.L. Chiswick). Churchill Livingstone, Edinburgh.

Herz, F. (1980) The Impact of Death and Serious Illness on the Family Life Cycle. In: *The Family Life Cycle,* (eds E. Carter & M. McGoldrick). Gardner, New York.

Hicks, C. (1992) Research in Midwifery: Are midwives their own worst enemies? *Midwifery,* **8**(1), 12–18.

Hicks, C. (1993) A Survey of Midwives' Attitudes to, and Involvement in, Research ... *Midwifery,* **9**(2), 51–62.

Hillier, S. (1981) Stresses, Strains and Smoking. *Nursing Mirror,* 12 February, 26–30.

Hingley, P. (1984) The Humane Face of Nursing. *Nursing Mirror,* 5 December, 19–22.

Hinton, J. (1977) *Dying.* Penguin Books Ltd., London.

Hockley, J. (1989) Caring for the Dying in Acute Hospitals. *Nursing Times,* **85**(39), 47–50.

Holland, S. (1987) Stress in Nursing 1 & 2. *Nursing Times,* **83**(21) and (30), 59–62 and 44–7.

Holland, J., Rmazanoglu, C., Scott, S., Sharpe, S. & Thomson, R. (1990) Sex, gender and power: Young women's sexuality in the shadow of AIDS. *Sociology of Health & Illness,* **12**(3), 337–50.

Horsley, A. (1990) The Neonatal Environment. *Paediatric Nursing,* February, pp 17–19.

House of Commons (1992) *Health Committee Second Report, Maternity Services.* HMSO, London.

Hu, D.J., Heyward, W.L., Byers, R.H. *et al.* (1992) HIV infection and breast-feeding: Policy implications through a decision analysis model. *AIDS,* **6**(12), 1505–13.

Hughes, P. (1986) *Solitary or Solitude: Views on the Management of Bereaved Mothers,* University of Wales, unpublished DipN Dissertation.

Hughes, P. (1987) The Management of Bereaved Mothers: What is Best? *Midwives Chronicle,* **100**(1195), 226–9.

Humble, S. & Unell, J. (1989) *Self-help in Health and Social Welfare: England and West Germany.* Routledge, London.

Hurme, H. (1991) Dimensions of the Grandparent Role in Finland. In: *The*

Psychology of Grandparenthood: An International Perspective, (ed. P.K. Smith). Routledge, London.

Hutchins, S.H. (1986) Stillbirth. In: Rando, T.A. *Parental Loss of a Child*. Research Press, Champaign, Illinois.

Iles, S. (1989) The loss of early pregnancy. In: *Psychological Aspects of Obstetrics and Gynaecology*, (ed. M.R. Oates), chapter 5. Baillière Tindall, London.

Illich, I. (1976) *Medical Nemesis: The Expropriation of Health*. Pantheon Books, New York.

International Planned Parenthood Convention (1991) Contraception and STDs. *IPPF Medical Bulletin*, **25**(5), 3–4.

Irvin, N.A., Kennell, J.H. & Klaus, M.H. (1982) Caring for the parents of an infant with a congenital malformation. In: Klaus, M. & Kennell, J. *Parent–Infant Bonding*, 2nd edn, Mosby, St Louis.

Jacques, C. (1992) Help on the Streets. *Nursing Times*, **28**(39), 24–6.

Jacques, N.C.S., Hawthorne-Amick, J.T. & Richards, M.P.M. (1983) Parents and the Support They Need. In: Davis, J.A., Richards, M.P.M. & Roberton, N.R.C. *Parent–Baby Attachment in Premature Infants*. Croom Helm Ltd., London.

Jeanty, P. & Romero, R. (1984) *Obstetrical Ultrasound*. McGraw Hill, New York.

Jemmott, L.S., Jemmott, J.B. III, & Cruz-Collins, M. (1992) Predicting AIDS patient care. *Nursing Research*, **41**(3), 172–7.

Jenkins, E. (1989) Handling loss: A systems framework. *Palliative Medicine*, **3**, 97–104.

Jick, T.D. (1983) Mixing Qualitative and Quantitative Methods: Triangulation in Action. In: *Qualitative Methodology*, (ed. J. van Maanen). Sage, Beverly Hills.

Johnson, S. (1984) Sexual Intimacy and Replacement Children After the Death of a Child. *Omega*, **15**, 109–18.

Johnstone, F.D., MacCallum, L., Brettle, R., Inglis, J.M., Peutherer, J.F. (1988) Does infection with HIV affect the outcome of pregnancy? *British Medical Journal*, **296**, 467.

Johnstone, F.D., Brettle, R.P., MacCallum, L.R., Mok, J., Peutherer, J.F. & Burns, S. (1990) Women's knowledge of their antibody state: its effect on their decision whether to continue the pregnancy. *British Medical Journal*, **300**, 23–4.

Jolly, J. (1987) *Missed Beginnings*. Lisa Sainsbury Foundation – Austen Cornish Publishers Ltd., London.

Jones, A. (1989) Managing the Invisible Grief. *Senior Nurse*, **9**(5), 26–7.

Kalish, R.A. (1985) *Death, Grief and Caring Relationships*, 2nd edn. Brooks Cole, California.

Kargar, I. (1990) Special Pregnancies. *Community Outlook*, June, pp. 12–18.

Kay, K. (1989) AIDS – A global concern. *Midwifery*, **5**(2), 84–5.

Kayiatos, R., Adams, J. & Gilman, B. (1984) The Arrival of a Rival. *Journal of Nurse-Midwifery*, **29**(3), 205–13.

Kell, P. & Barton, S. (1991) How do Women with HIV Present? *Maternal and Child Health*, **16**(11), 340–4.

Kellner, K.R. & Lake, M. (1986) Grief Counselling. In: Knuppel, R.A. & Drukker, J.E. *High Risk Pregnancy*. WB Saunders, Philadelphia.

Kennedy, J. & Edwards, S. (1993) HIV Infection in the Midwifery Setting. *Modern Midwife*, **3**(2) 25–7 & 29.

Kennell, J.H. & Klaus, M.H. (1982) Caring for the Parents of Premature or Sick Infants. In: Klaus, M.H. & Kennell, J.H. *Parent–Infant Bonding*, 2nd edn. Mosby, St Louis.

Kennell, J.H., Slyter, H. & Klaus, M.H. (1970) The Mourning Response of Parents to the Death of a Newborn Infant. *New England Journal of Medicine*, **283**(7), 344–9.

Kenyon, S. (1988) Support After Termination for Fetal Abnormality. *Midwives Chronicle*, **101**(1205), 190–1.

Kickbusch, I. (1989) Self-care in Health Promotion. *Social Science & Medicine*, **29**(2), 125–30.

Kirk, E. (1984) Psychological Effects and Management of Perinatal Loss. *American Journal of Obstetrics and Gynecology*, **149**, 45–61.

Kish, G. (1978) Notes on C. Grubb's Body Image Concerns of a Multipara in the Situation of Intrauterine Fetal Death. *Maternal Child Nursing Journal*, **7**, 111.

Klass, D. (1986) Bereaved Parents and the Compassionate Friends: Affiliation and Healing. *Omega*, **15**, 353–73.

Klass, D. & Shinners, B. (1983) Professional roles in a self-help group for the bereaved. *Omega*, **13**, 361–75.

Klaus, M.H., Jerauld, R., Kreger, N.C., McAlpine, W., Steffe, M. & Kennell, J.H. (1972) Maternal Attachment – importance of the first postpartum days. *New England Journal of Medicine*, **286**, 460–3.

Klaus, M. & Kennell, J. (1982a) An Evaluation of Interventions in the Premature Nursery. In: Davis, J.A., Richards, M.P.M. & Roberton, N.R.C. *Parent–Baby Attachment in Premature Infants*. Croom Helm Ltd., London.

Klaus, M. & Kennell, J. (1982b) *Parent–Infant Bonding*, 2nd edn. Mosby, St Louis.

Knight, B. & Hayes, R. (1981) *Self-help in the inner city*. London Voluntary Service Council.

Kohner, N. (1985) *Midwives and Stillbirth*. Royal College of Midwives/Health Education Council, London.

Kohner, N. & Henley, A. (1992) When a Baby Dies: *The Experience of Late Miscarriage, Stillbirth and Neonatal Death*. Pandora Press, London.

Kowalski, K.M. (1980) Managing Perinatal Loss. *Clinical Obstetrics and Gynecology*, **23**, 1113–23.

Kowalski, K.M. (1983) *A Bereaved Parent's Group: An Ethnographic Study*. University of Colorado, Boulder.

Kowalski, K.M. (1987) *Perinatal Loss and Bereavement*. In: Sonstegard, L., Kowalski, K.M. Jennings, B. *Women's Health: Crisis and Illness in Childbearing*. Grune & Stratton Inc., Orlando.

Kubler-Ross, E. (1970) *On Death and Dying*. Tavistock Publications Ltd., London.

Kuykendall, J. (1989) Death of a Child – The Worst Kept Secret Around. In *Death, Dying and Bereavement*, (ed. L. Sherr). Blackwell Scientific Publications, Oxford.

Kwast, B.E. (1991) Maternal Mortality: the magnitude and the causes. *Midwifery*, **7**(1), 4–7.

Lancaster, J. (1981) Impact of Intensive Care on the Parent–Child Relationship. In: Korones, S.B. *High Risk New Born Infants: The Basis for Intensive Nursing Care*. Mosby, St Louis.

Lapointe, N., Michaud, J. & Pekovich, D. (1985) Transplacental Transmission of HTLV III Virus. *New England Journal of Medicine*, **312**, 1325–6.

Laurence, K.M. (1989) Sequelae and Support for Termination Carried Out for Fetal Malformation. In: van Hall, E.V. & Everaerd, W. *The Free Woman: Women's Health in the 1990s*. Parthenon, Carnforth.

Laurent, C. (1993) A Sad Necessity. *Nursing Times*, **89**(13), 22.

Lazarus, R. (1976) *Patterns of Adjustment*. McGraw Hill, New York.

Leifer, A.D., Leiderman, P.H., Barnett, C.R. & Williams, J.A. (1972) Effects of Mother–Infant Separation on Material Attachment Behaviour. *Child Development*, **43**, 1203–18.

Leininger, M.M. (1985) *Qualitative Research Methods in Nursing*. Grune & Stratton Inc., Orlando.

Lendrum, S. & Syme, G. (1992) Gift of Tears: A Practical Approach to Loss and Bereavement Counselling, Tavistock/Routledge, London.

Leon, I.G. (1990) *When a Baby Dies: Psychotherapy for Pregnancy and Newborn Loss*. Yale University Press, London.

Leon, I.G. (1992) Commentary: Providing Versus Packaging Support for Bereaved Parents After Perinatal Loss. *Birth*, **19**(2), 89–91.

Leppert, P.C. & Pahlka, B.S. (1984) Grieving Characteristics After Spontaneous Abortion: A Management Approach. *Obstetrics and Gynaecology*, **64**, 119–22.

Lerum, C.W. & Lobiondo-Wood, G. (1989) The Relationship of Maternal Age, Quickening and Physical Symptoms of Pregnancy to the Development of Maternal–Fetal Attachment. *Birth*, **16**(1), 13–17.

Lewis, E. (1976) The Management of Stillbirth: Coping with an Unreality. *Lancet*, 7986 (ii), 619–20.

Lewis, E. (1979a) Mourning by the Family after a Stillbirth or Neonatal Death. *Archives of Disease in Childhood*, **54**, 303–6.

Lewis, E. (1979b) Inhibition of Mourning by Pregnancy: Psychopathology and Management. *British Medical Journal*, 6181, 27–8.

Lewis, E. & Bourne, S. (1989) Perinatal Death. In: *Psychological Aspects of Obstetrics and Gynaecology*, (ed. M. Oates). Baillière Tindall, London.

Lewis, E. & Bryan, E. (1988) Management of Perinatal Loss of a Twin. *British Medical Journal*, **297**, 1321–3.

Lewis, E. & Page, A. (1978) Failure to Mourn a Stillbirth. *British Journal of Medical Psychology*, **51**, 237–41.

Lewis, H. (1978) Nothing was said sympathy-wise. *Social Work Today*, **110**(45), 2479.

Lieberman, M.A. (1979) Analyzing Change Mechanisms in Groups. In: Lieberman, M.A., Borman, L.D., *et al. Self-help Groups for Coping With Crisis*. Jossey Bass, San Francisco.

Lieberman, M.A. & Bond, G.R. (1979) Problems in studying outcomes: In: Lieberman, M.A., Borman, L.D., *et al.* (1979) *Self-help Groups for Coping With Crisis*. Jossey-Bass, San Francisco.

Lieberman, M.A. & Gourash, N. (1979) Effects of Change Groups on the Elderly. In: Lieberman, M.A., Borman, L.D., *et al. Self-help Groups for Coping With Crisis.* Jossey Bass, San Francisco.

Lindemann, E. (1944) Symptomatology and Management of Acute Grief. *American Journal of Psychiatry,* **101**, 141–9.

Lindenfield, G. & Adams, R. (1984) *Problem solving through self-help groups.* Ilkely Self-help Associates, North Yorkshire.

Lipson, J.G. (1989) The Use of Self in Ethnographic Research. In: Morse, J.M. *Qualitative Nursing Research: A Contemporary Dialogue,* chapter 5. Rockville, Aspen.

Littlewood, J. (1992) *Aspects of Grief: Bereavement in Adult Life.* Tavistock/ Routledge, London.

Llewellyn-Jones, D. (1990) *Obstetrics and Gynaecology,* 5th edn, Faber & Faber Ltd., London.

Lloyd, J. & Laurence, K.M. (1985) Sequelae and Support After Termination of Pregnancy for Fetal Abnormality. *British Medical Journal,* **20**, 907–9.

Long, J. (1992) Grief and Loss in Childbirth. *Midwives Chronicle,* **105**(1250), 51–4.

Lovell, A. (1983) Women's Reactions to Late Miscarriage, Stillbirth and Perinatal Death. *Health Visitor,* **56**, 325–7.

Lovell, A. (1984) *A bereavement with a difference: A study of late miscarriage, stillbirth and perinatal death.* Sociology Department Occasional Paper 4, Polytechnic of the South Bank, London.

Lovell, H., Bokoula, C., Misra, S. & Speight, N. (1986) Mothers' Reactions to Perinatal Death. *Nursing Times,* **82**(46), 40–2.

Lugton, J. (1989) *Communicating with Dying People and their Relatives.* Lisa Sainsbury Foundation – Austen Cornish Publishers Ltd., London.

Lumley, J. (1980) The Image of the Fetus in the First Trimester. *Birth and the Family Journal,* **7**, 5–12.

Lumley, J. (1990) Through a glass darkly: Ultrasound and prenatal bonding. *Birth,* **17**(4), 214–7.

Lumley, L.J. (1979) The Development of Maternal Fetal Bonding in the First Pregnancy. In: *Emotion and Reproduction,* (eds L. Carena & L. Zichella), 5th International Congress of Psychosomatic Obstetrics and Gynaecology. Academic Press, London.

Lyall, J. (1992) Outreaching. *Nursing Times,* **88**(27), 16–17.

McCaffery, M. (1979) *Nursing Management of the Patient in Pain.* Lippincott, New York.

McCarthy, K.H., Johnson, M.A. & Studd, J.W.W. (1992) Antenatal HIV Testing. *British Journal of Obstetrics and Gynaecology,* **99**(11), 867–8.

McHaffie, H.E. (1988) *A Prospective Study to Identify Critical Factors Which Indicate Mothers' Readiness to Care for their VLBW Babies at Home.* Unpublished PhD Thesis, University of Edinburgh.

McHaffie, H.E. (1991) *A Study of Support for Families with a VLBW Baby.* University of Edinburgh Nursing Research Unit.

McHaffie, H.E. (1992) Social Support in the NNICU. *Journal of Advanced Nursing,* **17**, 279–87.

McNeil, J.N. (1986) Communicating With Surviving Children. In: Rando, T.A. *Parental Loss of a Child,* Research Press, Champaign, Illinois.

McNeill-Taylor, L. (1983) *Living With Loss – A Book for the Widowed.* Fontana Press, Glasgow.

Macintyre, S. (1975) *Decision-making processes following premarital conception.* Unpublished PhD Thesis, University of Glasgow.

Mallinson, G. (1989) Life Crises; When a Baby Dies. *Nursing Times*, **85**(9), 31–4.

Mandelbaum, D.E. (1959) Social Uses of Funeral Rites. In: Feifel, H. *The Meaning of Death.* McGraw-Hill, New York.

Mandell, F. & Wolfe, L.C. (1975) Sudden Infant Death Syndrome and Subsequent Pregnancy. *Pediatrics*, **56**(5), 774–6.

Mander, R. (1992a) The Control of Pain in Labour. *Journal of Clinical Nursing*, **1**, 219–23.

Mander, R. (1992b) See How They Learn: Experience as the Basis of Practice. *Nurse Education Today*, **12**, 11–8.

Mander, R. (1992c) Seeking Approval for Research Access: The gatekeepers' role in facilitating a study of the care of the relinquishing mother. *Journal of Advanced Nursing*, **17**(12), 1460–4.

Mander, R. (1992d) *Research Report: Midwives' Care of the Relinquishing Mother.* The Iolanthe Trust, London.

Mander, R. (1993) Who chooses the choices? *Modern Midwife*, **3**(1), 23–5.

Mander, R. & Whyte, D.W. (1985) Assisted Reproduction: Setting the Limits? *Midwifery*, **1**, 232–9.

Marris, P. (1986) *Loss and Change.* Routledge/Kegan Paul International Ltd., London.

Martin, J. (1993) Doctor's Mask on Pain. In: Dickenson, D. & Johnson, M. *Death, Dying and Bereavement.* Open University and Sage, London.

Menning, B.E. (1982) The Psychosocial Impact of Infertility. *The Nursing Clinics of North America*, **17**(1), 155–63.

Menzies, I.E.P. (1961) The functioning of social systems as a defence against anxiety. In: Macguire, J. *Threshold to Nursing*, Bell & Hyman Ltd., London.

Miller, E. & Webb, B. (1988) *The Nature of Effective Self-help Support in Different Contexts.* Tavistock Institute of Human Relations, London.

Moore, M.L. (1981) *Newborn Family and Nurse.* W.B. Saunders, Philadelphia.

Morlat, P., Parmeix, P., Douard, D. *et al.* (1992) Women and HIV infection: A cohort study of 483 HIV infected women in Bordeaux 1985–1991. *AIDS*, **6**(10), 1187–94.

Morrin, N. (1983) As Great a Loss. *Nursing Mirror*, **156**(7), 33.

Morse, J.M., Bottorff, J., Anderson, G., O'Brien, B. & Solberg, S. (1992) Beyond Empathy: Expanding expressions of caring. *Journal of Advanced Nursing*, **17**, 809–21.

Murdoch, D.R. & Darlow, B.A. (1984) Handling During Neonatal Intensive Care. *Archives of Disease in Childhood*, **59**, 957–61.

Murgatroyd, S. & Woolfe, R. (1982) *Coping with Crisis: Understanding and helping people in need.* Harper & Row, London.

Murray, J. & Callan, V.J. (1988) Predicting Adjustment to Perinatal Death. *British Journal of Medical Psychology*, **61**, 237–44.

Mussen, P.H., Janeway, J., Kagan, J. & Huston, A.C. (1990) *Child Personality and Development.* Harper & Row, New York.

Nelson, D., Heitman, R. & Jennings, C. (1986) Effects of Tactile Stimulation on Premature Weight Gain. *Journal of Obstetric Gynècologic and Neonatal Nursing,* May/Jun, 262–7.

Nichols, J.A. (1984) Illegitimate Mourners. In: *Children and Death: Perspectives and Challenges.* Symposium, Akron, Ohio.

Nichols, J.A. (1986) Newborn Death. In: Rando, T.A. *Parental Loss of a Child.* Research Press, Champaign, Illinois.

Niven, C.A. (1992) *Psychological Care for Families: Before, During and After Birth.* Butterworth–Heinemann, Oxford.

Norman, S., Studd, J. & Johnson, M. (1990) HIV infection in Women. *British Medical Journal,* **301**, 1231–2.

Oakley, A., McPherson, A. & Roberts, H. (1984) *Miscarriage.* Penguin Books, London.

Oglethorpe, R.J.L. (1989) Parenting After Perinatal Bereavement – A Review of the Literature. *Journal of Reproductive and Infant Psychology,* **7**(4), 227–44.

Osterweis, M., Solomon, F. & Green, M. (1984) *Bereavement: Reactions Consequences and Care.* Committee for the Study of the Health Consequences of the Stress of Bereavement, Washington DC, National Academy Press.

Panos Dossier (1990) *Triple Jeopardy.* Panos Institute, Budapest.

Parkes, C.M. (1972) *Bereavement.* International Universities Press, New York.

Parkes, C.M. (1976) *Bereavement: Studies of Grief in Adult Life.* Penguin Books, Harmondsworth.

Parkes, C.M. (1980) Bereavement Counselling: Does it Work? *British Medical Journal,* **282**(4), 3–6.

Parrish, S. (1980) Letting go. *Canadian Nurse,* **76**(3), 34–7.

Parse, R.R., Coyne, A.B. & Smith, M.J. (1985) *Nursing Research: Qualitative Methods.* Brady Communications, Bowie, Maryland.

Parsons, T. (1951) *The Social System.* The Free Press, Glencoe, Illinois.

Pearson, A., & Vaughan, B. (1989) *Nursing Models for Practice,* Heinemann Medical Books, Oxford.

Penson, J.M. (1990) *Bereavement: A Guide for Nurses,* Harper & Row, London.

Penticuff, J.H. (1992) The Impact of the Child Abuse Amendments on Nursing Staff and their Care of Handicapped Newborns. In: Caplan, A.L., Blank, R.H. & Merrick, J.C. *Compelled Compassion: Government Intervention in the Treatment of Critically Ill Newborns.* Human Press, Totowa, New Jersey.

Peplau, H. (1976) Anxiety. In *Childbearing: A Nursing Perspective,* (eds A.L. Clark & D. Affonso). F.A. Davis & Co., Philadelphia.

Peppers, L. & Knapp, R. (1982) Motherhood and Mourning. Praeger, New York.

Peppers, L.G. & Knapp, R.J. (1980) Maternal Reactions to Involuntary Fetal/ Infant Death, *Psychiatry,* **43**, 155–9.

Perakyla, A. & Bor, R. (1990) Interactional problems of addressing 'dreaded issues' in HIV counselling. *AIDS Care,* **2**(4), 325–37.

Peretz, D. (1970) Reactions to Loss. In: *Loss and Grief: Psychological Management in Medical Practice*, (eds B. Schoènberg, A.C. Karr, D. Peretz & A.H. Kutscher). Columbia University Press.

Perry, S. (1993) Personal Communcation.

Phoenix, A. (1990) Black Women and the Maternity Services. In: Garcia, J., Kilpatrick, R. & Richards, M. *The Politics of Maternity Care: Services for Childbearing Women in Twentieth-Century Britain*. Oxford University Press.

Piaget, J. (1952) *The Origins of Intelligence in Children*. International University Press, New York.

Pine, V.R. & Brauer, C. (1986) Parental Grief: A Synthesis of Theory Research and Intervention. In: Rando, T.A. *Parental Loss of a Child*. Research Press, Champaign, Illinois.

Polak, P.R., Egan, D., Lee, J.H., Vandenburgh, R.H. & Williams, W.V. (1975) Prevention in Mental Health: A Controlled Study. *American Journal of Psychiatry*, **132**, 146–9.

Prior, L. (1993) The Social Distribution of Sentiments. In: Dickenson, D. & Johnson, M. *Death, Dying and Bereavement*. Open University and Sage, London.

Queenan, J. (1978) The Ultimate Defeat. *Contemporary Obstetrics and Gynaecology*, **11**, 7.

Quirk, T.S. (1979) Crisis Theory, Grief Theory and Related Psychosocial Factors: The Framework for Intervention. *Journal of Nurse-Midwifery*, **24**, 13.

Rajan, L. & Oakley, A., (1993) No pills for the heartache: the importance of social support for women who suffer pregnancy loss. *Journal of Reproductive and Infant Psychology*, **11**(2), 75–88.

Rando, T.A. (1986a) Unique Issues and Impact. In: Rando, T.A. *Parental Loss of a Child*. Research Press, Champaign, Illinois.

Rando, T.A. (1986b) Individual and Couples Treatment Following the Death of a Child. In: Rando, T.A. *Parental Loss of a Child*. Research Press, Champaign, Illinois.

Rando, T.A. (1986c) *Parental Loss of a Child*. Research Press, Champaign Illinois.

Raphael, B. (1977) Preventive Interventions with the Recently Bereaved. *Archives of General Psychiatry*, **34**, 1450–4.

Raphael, B. (1983) *The Anatomy of Bereavement*. Basic Books, New York.

Raphael, B. (1984a) *The Anatomy of Bereavement: A handbook for the caring professions*. Unwin Hyman, London.

Raphael, B. (1984b) Personal Disaster. *Australian and New Zealand Journal of Psychiatry*, **15**, 183–98.

Raphael-Leff, J. (1991) *Psychological Processes of Childbearing*. Chapman & Hall, London.

Rapoport, C. (1981) Helping Parents When Their Newborn Infants Die: Social Work Implications. *Social Work in Health Care*, **6**(3), 57–67.

Reading, A.E. (1989) The Measurement of Fetal Attachment Over the Course of Pregnancy. In: van Hall, E.V. & Everaerd, W. *The Free Woman: Women's Health in the 1990s*. Parthenon, Carnforth.

Reid, M. (1990) Prenatal diagnosis and screening. In: Garcia, J., Kilpatrick, R. &

Richards, M. *The Politics of Maternity Care: Services for Childbearing Women in Twentieth-Century Britain*, chapter 16. Oxford University Press.

Richards, M.P.M. (1983) Parent–Child Relationships: Some General Considerations. In: Davis, J.A., Richards, M.P.M. & Roberton, N.R.C. *Parent–Baby Attachment in Premature Infants*. Croom Helm, London.

Richards, M.P.M. (1987) The Withdrawal of Treatment from Newborn Infants. *Midwives Information and Resource Service Information Pack*, **5**, August.

Richards, M.P.M. (1989) Social and Ethical Problems of Fetal Diagnosis and Screening. *Journal of Reproductive & Infant Psychology*, **7**(2), 171–85.

Richardson, A. & Goodman, M. (1983) *Self-help and Social Care: Mutual Aid Organisations in Practice*. London Policy Studies Institute.

Ridley, S. (1993) Psychological Defence Mechanisms and Coping Strategies. In: Dickenson, D. & Johnson, M. *Death, Dying and Bereavement*. Open University and Sage, London.

Roberts, F.B. (1977) *Perinatal Nursing: Care of Newborns and their Families*. McGraw-Hill, New York.

Roberts, H. (1989) A Baby or the Products of Conception: Lay and Professional Perspectives on Miscarriage. In: van Hall, E.V. & Everaerd, W. *The Free Woman: Women's Health in the 1990s*. Parthenon, Carnforth.

Robertson, R.J., Skidmore, C.A., Roberts, J.J.K. & Elton, R.A. (1990) Progression to AIDS in Intravenous Drug Users, Cofactors and Survival, *VI International Conference on AIDS*, San Francisco, June 1990, (Abstract ThC649).

Robinson, D. & Henry, S. (1977) *Self-help and Health: Mutual Aid for Modern Problems*. Martin Robertson, London.

Roch, S. (1987) Sharing the Grief. *Nursing Times*, **83**(14) 52–3.

Roll, S., Millen, L. & Backlund, B. (1986) Solomon's Mothers: Mourning in Mothers who Relinquish their Children for Adoption. In: Rando, T.A. *Parental Loss of a Child*. Research Press, Champaign, Illinois.

Rose, X. (1990) *Widow's Journey: A Return to Living*. Souvenir Press, London.

Roth, C. & Brierley, J. (1990) HIV Infection – A Midwifery Perspective. In: Alexander, J., Levy, V. & Roch, S. *Intra Partum Care*. Macmillan Education, Basingstoke.

Rothman, B.K. (1986) *The Tentative Pregnancy: Prenatal Diagnosis and the Future of Motherhood*. Pandora Press, London.

Rothman, B.K. (1990) Commentary: Women Feel Social and Economic Pressures to Abort Abnormal Fetuses. *Birth*, **17**(2), 81.

Rowe, J., Clyman, R., Green, C. *et al.* (1978) Follow-up of Families who Experienced a Perinatal Death. *Pediatrics*, **62**(2), 166–9.

Rubin, R. (1967) Attachment of the Maternal Role. *Nursing Research*, **16**, 237–45.

Rubin, R. (1975) Maternal Tasks in Pregnancy. *Maternal Child Nursing Journal*, **4**, 143.

Rynearson, E.K. (1987) Psychotherapy of Pathologic Grief: Revisions and Limitations. *Psychiatric Clinics of North America*, **10**(3), 487–99.

Sandbank, A. (1988) *Twins and the Family*. Arrow Books, London.

SANDS (1991) *Miscarriage, stillbirth and neonatal death: guidelines for professionals*. Stillbirth and Neonatal Death Society, London.

Selye, H. (1956) *The Stress of Life*. McGraw Hill, New York.

Selye, H. (1980) Stress and a Holistic View of Health for the Nursing Profession. In: *Living with Stress and Promoting Well-being*, (eds K. Claus & J. Bailey). Mosby, St Louis.

Schaffer, R. (1977) *Mothering: The Developing Child*. Fontana, Glasgow.

Schatz, W.H. (1986) The Grief of Fathers. In: Rando, T.A. *Parental Loss of a Child*. Research Press, Champaign, Illinois.

Schiff, H. (1979) *The Bereaved Parent*. Souvenir Press, London.

Sheard, T. (1984) Dealing with the Nurse's Grief. *Nursing Forum*, **21**(1), 43–5.

Sherr, L. (1989a) AIDS. In: *Death, Dying and Bereavement*, (ed. L. Sherr), chapter 12. Blackwell Scientific Publications, Oxford.

Sherr, L. (1989b) Death of a Baby. In: *Death, Dying and Bereavement*, (ed. L. Sherr). Blackwell Scientific Publications, Oxford.

Sherr, L. (ed.) (1989c) *Death, Dying and Bereavement*. Blackwell Scientific Publications, Oxford.

Sherr, L. (1991) *HIV and AIDS in Mothers and Babies*. Blackwell Scientific Publications, Oxford.

Sherr, L. & George, H. (1988) *AIDS and Staff Stress*. Abstracts, Psychology and Health International, British Psychological Society, London.

Sherr, L. & George, H. (1989) Loss and the Human Immunodeficiency Virus. In: *Death, Dying and Bereavement*, (ed. L. Sherr), chapter 11. Blackwell Scientific Publications, Oxford.

Sherratt, D. (1987) What Do You Say? *Midwives Chronicle*, **100**(1195), 235–6.

Simmons, M. (1992) Helping Children Grieve. *Nursing Times*, **88**(50), 30–2.

Sluckin, W., Herbert, M. & Sluckin, A. (1983) *Maternal Bonding*. Blackwell Scientific Publications, Oxford.

Smialek, Z. (1978) Observations on Immediate Reactions of Families to Sudden Infant Death. *Pediatrics*, **62**(2), 160–5.

Smith, M.S. (1991b) An Evolutionary Perspective on Grandparent–Grandchild Relationships. In: *The Psychology of Grandparenthood: An International Perspective*, (ed. P.K. Smith). Routledge, London.

Smith, P.K. (1991a) Introduction: The Study of Grandparenthood. In: *The Psychology of Grandparenthood: An International Perspective*, (ed. P.K. Smith). Routledge, London.

Solkoff, N. Yasse, S. Weintraub, D. & Blase, D. (1969) Effects of Handling on the Subsequent Development of Premature Infants. *Developmental Psychology*, **1**, 765–8.

Solnit, A.J. & Stark, M.H. (1961) Mourning and the Birth of a Defective Child. *Psychoanalytical Study of the Child*, **16**, 523–37.

Sorosky, A.D., Baran, A. & Pannor, R. (1984) *The Adoption Triangle*. Anchor, New York.

Spinks, P. & Michaelson, J. (1989) A Comparison of the Ward Environment in a SCBU and a Children's Orthopaedic Ward. *Journal of Reproductive and Infant Psychology*, **7**(1), 47–50.

Stack, J. (1982) *Reproductive Casualties*. Perinatal Press, New York.

Stainton, M.C. (1990) Parents' Awareness of Their Unborn Infant in the Third Trimester. *Birth*, **17**(2), 92–6.

Standish, E. (1982) The Loss of a Baby. *Lancet*, **1**, 611–12.

Statham, H. & Dimavicius, J. (1992) Commentary: How Do You Give the Bad News to Parents? *Birth*, **19**(2), 103–4.

Stephenson, J. (1986) Grief of Siblings. In: Rando, T.A. *Parental Loss of a Child*. Research Press, Champaign, Illinois.

Stern, P.N. (1980) Grounded Theory Methodology: Its Uses and Processes. *Image*, **12**(1), 20–23.

Stray-Pedersen, B. & Stray-Pedersen, S. (1984) Etiologic factors and subsequent reproductive performance in 195 couples with a prior history of habitual abortion. *American Journal of Obstetrics and Gynecology*, **148**(2), 140–6.

Stroebe, W. & Stroebe, M.S. (1987) *Bereavement and Health: The Psychological and Physical Consequences of Partner Loss*. Cambridge University Press.

Tom-Johnson, C. (1990) Talking Through Grief. *Nursing Times*, **86**(1), 44–6.

Tschudin, V. (1982) *Counselling Skills for Nurses*. Baillière Tindall, London.

Tschudin, V. (1985) Warding off a Crisis. *Nursing Times*, **81**(38), 45–6.

Tudehope, D.I., Iredell, J., Rodgers, D. & Gunn, A. (1986) Neonatal Death: Grieving Families. *The Medical Journal of Australia*, **144**, 290–1.

Turrill, S. (1992) Supported Positioning in Intensive Care. *Paediatric Nursing*, **4**(4), 24–7.

Van Maanen, J. (1982) Introduction. In: Van Maanen, J. Dabb, S. & Faulkner, S. *Varieties of Qualitative Research*. Sage, Beverly Hills.

Veksner, S. (1993) Real lives: Bud medicine. *The Guardian Weekend*, 17 April, pp. 18–20.

Videka, L.M. (1979) Psychosocial Adaptation in a Medical Self-help Group. In: Lieberman, M.A., Borman, L.D. *et al. Self-help Groups for Coping With Crisis*. Jossey Bass, San Francisco.

Videka-Sherman, L.M. (1982) Coping with the death of a child. *American Journal of Orthopsychiatry*, **51**(4), 699–703.

Vogel, H.P. & Knox, E.G. (1975) Reproductive Patterns after Stillbirth and Early Infant Death. *Journal of Biosocial Science*, **7**, 103–11.

Walker, R. (1992) One From the Heart. *Nursing Times*, **88**(1), 27.

Waller, D.A., Todres, D., Cassem, N.H. & Anderten, A. (1979) Coping with Poor Prognosis in the Paediatric ICU: The Cassandra Prophecy. *American Journal of Diseases in Childhood*, **133**, 1121–5.

Wallston, K.A. & Wallston, B.S. (1981) Health locus of control scales. In: Lefcourt, H.M. *Research with the locus of control construct*. Academic Press, New York.

Ward Davies, S. (1990) Women and AIDS: putting the picture in perspective: the facts. *The Guardian*, 29 November, p21.

Watson, N. (1993) Personal Communication.

Werner, N.P. & Conway, A.E. (1990) Caregiver contacts experienced by premature infants in a NNICU. *Maternal–Child Nursing Journal*, **19**(1), 21–43.

Wesson, N. (1989) Personal Communication. In: Roberts, H. van Hall, E.V. &

Everaerd, W. *The Free Woman: Women's Health in the 1990s*, Parthenon, Carnforth.

White, M.P., Reynolds, B. & Evans, T.J. (1984) Handling of Death in SCUs and Parental Grief. *British Medical Journal*, **289**, 167–9.

WHO (1983) *Self-help and health in Europe*, World Health Organisation Regional Office for Europe, Copenhagen.

Whyte, D.A. (1989) *The Experience of Families Caring for a Child with Cystic Fibrosis: A Nursing Response*. Unpublished PhD Thesis, University of Edinburgh.

Williams, W.V. & Polak, P.R. (1979) Follow-up research in primary prevention. *Journal of Clinical Psychiatry*, **35**(1), 35–45.

Wilson, A.L., Lawrence, J.F., Stevens, D.C. & Soule, D.J. (1982) The Death of a Newborn Twin. *Pediatrics*, **70**(4), 487–91.

Wilson, H. (1985) *Research in Nursing*. Addison Wesley, California.

Wilson, J. & Breedon, P. (1990) Universal Precautions. *Nursing Times*, **86**(37), 67–70.

Winkler, R. & Van Keppel, M. (1984) *Relinquishing Mothers in Adoption*. Melbourne Institute of Family Studies Monograph 3, Australia.

Wolff, J.R., Nielson, P.E. & Schiller, P. (1970) The Emotional Reaction to Stillbirth. *American Journal of Obstetrics and Gynecology*, **108**(1), 73–7.

Wolke, D. (1987a) Environmental and Developmental Neonatology. *Journal of Reproductive and Infant Psychology*, **5**(1), 17–42.

Wolke, D. (1987b) Environmental Neonatology. *Archives of Diseases in Childhood*, **62**, 87–8.

Woodward, S., Pope, A., Robson, W.J. & Hagan, O. (1985) Bereavement Counselling After Sudden Death. *British Medical Journal*, **290**, 363–5.

Woollett, A. & Dosanjh-Matwala, N. (1990) Post natal care: The attitudes and experiences of Asian women in East London. *Midwifery*, **6**(4), 178–84.

Worden, J.W. (1992) *Grief Counselling and Grief Therapy: A Handbook for the Mental Health Practitioner*, 2nd edn. Routledge, London.

Wright, B. (1991) *Sudden Death: Intervention Skills for the Caring Professions*. Churchill Livingstone, Edinburgh.

Yates, D.W., Ellison, G. & McGuiness, S. (1993) Care of the Suddenly Bereaved. In: Dickenson, D. & Johnson, M. *Death, Dying and Bereavement*. Open University and Sage, London.

Yates, S.A. (1972) Stillbirth: What a Staff can do. *American Journal of Nursing*, **72**, 1592–4.

Zeanah, C.H., Carr, S. & Wolk, S. (1990) Fetal Movements and the Imagined Baby of Pregnancy: Are They Related? *Journal of Reproductive and Infant Psychology*, **8**(1), 23–36.

Further Reading

Benfield, D.G. Leib, S.A. & Vollman, J.H. (1978) Grief Response of Parents to Neonatal Death and Parent Participation in Deciding Care, *Pediatrics*, **6**(2), 171–6.

Bourne, S. (1983) Psychological Impact of Stillbirth. *The Practitioner*, **227**, 533–9.

Bowlby, J. (1979) *The Making and Breaking of Affectional Bonds*. Tavistock Publications, London.

Cook, A.S. & Oltjenbruns, K.A. (1989) *Dying and Grieving: Lifespan and Family Perspectives*. Holt Rhinehart & Winston, New York.

Couldrick, A. (1992) Optimising Bereavement Outcomes: Reading the Road Ahead. *Social Science and Medicine*, **35**(12), 1521–3.

Dickenson, D. & Johnson, M. (eds) (1993) *Death, Dying and Bereavement*. Open University and Sage, London.

Dyregrov, A. (1988) The Loss of a Child: The Sibling's Perspective. In: *Motherhood and Mental Illness 2: Causes and Consequences*, (eds R. Kumar & N. Brockington). Wright, London.

Forrest, G. (1989) Care of the Bereaved after Perinatal Death. In: Chalmers, I., Enkin, M. & Keirse, M.J.N.C. *Effective Care in Pregnancy and Childbirth*, **2**. Oxford University Press.

Kennell, J.H., Jerauld, R., Wolfe, H., Chester, D., Kreger, N.C., McAlpine, W., Steffa, M. & Klaus, M.H. (1974) Maternal Behaviour One Year After Early and Extended Post-partum Contact. *Developmental Medicine and Child Neurology*, **16**, 172–9.

Kitson, A. (1990) *Quality Patient Care: The Dynamic Standard Setting System*. Royal College of Nursing, London.

Klaus, M. & Kennell, J. (1982) *Parent–Infant Bonding*, 2nd edn. Mosby, St Louis.

Klein, M. (1963) *Our Adult World and Other Essays*. Heinemann Medical Books, Oxford.

Leon, I.G. (1990) *When a Baby Dies: Psychotherapy for Pregnancy and Newborn Loss*. Yale University Press, London.

Lewis, E. & Bourne, S. (1989) Perinatal Death. In: *Psychological Aspects of Obstetrics and Gynaecology*, (ed. M. Oates). Baillière Tindall, London.

Littlewood, J. (1992) *Aspects of Grief: Bereavement in Adult Life*. Tavistock/ Routledge, London.

Loudun, I. (1992) *Death in Childbirth: An International Study of Maternal Care and Maternal Mortality 1800–1950*. Clarendon Press, Oxford.

Luthert, J.M. & Robinson, L. (1993) *Manual of Standards of Care*. Blackwell Scientific Publications, Oxford.

Marris, P. (1986) *Loss and Change*. Routledge/Kegan Paul, London.

News (1992) The Risk of Women Dying as a Result of Pregnancy. *Birth*, **19**(3), 171.

Oakley, A., McPherson, A. & Roberts, H. (1990) *Miscarriage*. Penguin Books, London.

Oglethorpe, R.J.L. (1989) Parenting After Perinatal Bereavement – A Review of the Literature. *Journal of Reproductive and Infant Psychology*, **7**(4), 227–44.

Osterweis, M., Solomon, F. & Green, M. (1984) *Bereavement: Reactions, Consequences and Care*. Committee for the Study of the Health Consequences of the Stress of Bereavement, Washington DC, National Academy Press.

Parkes, C.M. (1979) Grief. In: *Terminal Care*, (ed. D. Doyle). Churchill Livingstone, Edinburgh.

Poovan, P., Fesehatsion, K. & Kwast, B.E. (1990) A Maternity Waiting Home Reduces Obstetric Catastrophes. *World Health Forum*, **11**(4), 440–5.

Rando, T.A. (1986) *Parental Loss of a Child*. Research Press, Champaign, Illinois.

Raphael, B. (1984) *The Anatomy of Bereavement: A handbook for the caring professions*. Unwin Hyman, London.

Richards, M.P.M. (1983) Parent–Child Relationships: Some General Considerations. In: Davis, J.A., Richards, M.P.M. & Roberton, N.R.C. *Parent–Baby Attachment in Premature Infants*. Croom Helm, London.

Sherr, L. (ed.) (1989) *Death, Dying and Bereavement*. Blackwell Scientific Publications, Oxford.

Snowley, G.D. & Nicklin, P.J. (1989) *Objectives for Care: Specifying Standards for Clinical Nursing*. Austen Cornish Publishers, London.

Worden, J.W. (1992) *Grief Counselling and Grief Therapy: A Handbook for the Mental Health Practitioner*, 2nd edn. Routledge, London.

Appendix
Useful Addresses

These addresses were correct at the time of writing. Details have kindly been provided by the staff of the organisations.

Bereavement care

CRUSE – Bereavement Care
126 Sheen Road
Richmond
Surrey
TW9 1UR
081 940 4818

Cruse Bereavement Line 081 332 7227 which provides a direct link to a counsellor Monday – Friday 09.30–17.00.
Cruse offers free help to all bereaved people through its 194 local branches, by providing both individual and group counselling, and opportunities for social contact and practical advice. A list of related publications and a newsletter are also available.

LABS (The London Association of Bereavement Services)
London Voluntary Sector Resource Centre
356 Holloway Road
London
N7 6PN
071 700 8134 (Answerphone outside office hours)

LABS is an umbrella organisation for bereavement services in the Greater London Area, which provides counselling and support for those whose relatives or friends have died. Callers are referred to their nearest local service or to other organisations. In-service training is provided for volunteers and professionals. LABS acts as an advisory body for those seeking to establish a service.

The Samaritans
The General Office of the Samaritans
10 The Grove
Slough
Berkshire
SL1 1PQ

Administrative office: 0753 532713
Local telephone numbers are in telephone directories.
Aims: to offer emotional support to anyone passing through a period of personal crisis, and who is suicidal or at risk of becoming suicidal, through befriending which is confidential and easily available 24 hours a day.

Sudden Infant Death Syndrome (SIDS)

Foundation for the Study of Infant Deaths
15 Belgrave Square
London
SW1X 8QB
071 235 0965

Aims: fundraising for research into causes/prevention of SIDS
support bereaved parents
information source for parents, professionals and public.

The Scottish Cot Death Trust
Royal Hospital for Sick Children
Yorkhill
Glasgow
G3 8SJ
041 357 3946

Aims: to raise substantial sums of money to initiate and fund research into the causes and the prevention of cot death
to extend and improve the support given to bereaved families including supplying breathing monitors for their subsequent babies
to educate the public about cot death through information leaflets, the media and meetings.

HIV/AIDS

Body Positive
The Body Positive Centre
51B Philbeach Gdns
Earls Court
London SW5 9EB
071 835 1045

Helpline 19.00–22.00 daily 071 373 9124
Aims: to provide emotional support, practical help and information for people affected by HIV/AIDS
Activities: a helpline
a newsletter
a drop-in centre

training weekends
hospital and prison visiting
a hardship fund
support groups for: women
young people
people in prison
newly diagnosed people
a UK-wide national network.

London Lighthouse
111–117 Lancaster Road
London
W11 1QT
071 792 1200

Aims: counselling and social support for people affected by HIV/AIDS.
Activities: creative and complementary therapies
community services
day care
residential, respite, convalescent and palliative care
education and training.

Positively Women
5 Sebastian Street
London
EC1V 0HE
071 490 5515

Helpline 12.00–14.00 daily 071 490 2327
Aims: to protect the health of women by counselling and support
to serve women who have AIDS, HIV or any associated conditions
to advance relevant education and research
to give advice, assistance and other charitable activities.

Terence Higgins Trust
52–54 Grays Inn Road
London
WC1X 8JU

Helpline 12.00–22.00 daily 071 242 1010
Legal line 19.00–22.00 Wednesday 071 405 2381
Aims: anti-HIV education
counselling service
buddying scheme
practical help
pressure group activities

Miscarriage

Miscarriage Association
c/o Clayton Hospital
Northgate
Wakefield
West Yorkshire
WF1 3JS
0924 200799

Aims: local self-help groups
national helpline
information for affected mothers
consciousness-raising
good practice guide for professionals.

Euthanasia

Voluntary Euthanasia Society
13 Prince of Wales Terrace
London
W8 5PG
071 937 7770

Aims: to campaign to change the law to permit the right to die with dignity.

Perinatal loss

Blisslink/Nippers
Janet Palmer
PO Box 1553
Wedmore
Somerset
BS28 4LZ
0934 713630

Special Memories – Part of Blisslink/Nippers, the national support group for parents of special care babies. Special Memories offers support for parents whose babies die in a special care baby unit, or after discharge from SCBU. Newsletter, leaflets and telephone support.

The Compassionate Friends
53 North Street
Bristol
BS3 1EN

Helpline 0272 539 639
A nationwide self-help organisation of parents whose child of any age, including adult, has died from any cause. Personal and group support. Quarterly newsletter, postal library and a range of leaflets. Befriending not counselling.

SANDS (Stillbirth and Neonatal Death Society)
28 Portland Place
London
W1N 4DE
071 436 7940

Helpline 071 436 5881
Aims: to provide support to parents who have lost a baby during late pregnancy or around the time of birth.
There is a network of support groups throughout the country and a wide range of publications, which may be obtained from the address given above.

Relinquishment

Family Care
21 Castle Street
Edinburgh
EH2 3DN
031 225 6441

A voluntary social work agency and approved adoption society, which offers an adoption enquiry and counselling service and also help for people with fertility problems.

National Organisation for the Counselling of Adoptees and Parents (NORCAP)
3 New High Street
Headington
Oxford
OX3 7AJ
0865 750554

Aims: to provide support, guidance and sympathetic understanding to adult adoptees and their birth and adoptive parents.
Activities: telephone counselling service; advice on searching and research service; intermediary role for those seeking renewed contact; liaison with other formal agencies.

NORCAP Natural Parents Support Group (NPSG) – for Birth Parents
Jan Hanmer
3 Alder Grove
Normanton
West Yorkshire
WF6 1LF
0924 894076

Post-Adoption Centre
5 Torriano Mews
Torriano Avenue
London
NW5 2RZ
071 284 0555

Aims: to provide counselling and family work for anybody involved in an adoption. This of course includes birth mothers who have lost their children through adoption.

Special groups

ISSUE (The National Fertility Association) (England, Wales and Ireland)
509 Aldridge Road
Great Barr
Birmingham
B44 8NA
021 344 4414

ISSUE (Scotland)
21 Castle Street
Edinburgh
EH2 3DN
031 225 2464

ISSUE is a national self-help organisation which provides information, support and representation to people with fertility difficulties and those who work with them.

Jewish Bereavement Counselling Service
c/o Visitation Committee
Woburn House
Tavistock Square
London
WC1H 0EZ
081 349 0839 or 071 387 4300 x227

Aims: to provide bereavement counselling and support by trained voluntary counsellors to members of the Jewish community who live in NW and SW London and the London Borough of Redbridge.

PROPES (Parents Recognition of Paediatric Errors)
Iatrogenic Centre
56 Southland Drive
West Cross
Swansea
SA3 5RJ
0792 403593

SATFA (Support Around Termination For Abnormality)
29–30 Soho Square
London
W1V 6JB
071 287 3753

Helpline 071 439 6124
Aims: to help parents who discover their unborn baby is abnormal
        to provide information and individual and group support
        to work with professionals to improve parents' care.

CARE
The Scottish Association for Care and Support after the Diagnosis of Fetal Abnormality
c/o Carol Reid
36 Canmore Place
Stewarton
Ayrshire
KA3 5PS
0560 483310

A voluntary organisation comprising a network of mutual help groups to provide support after termination for fetal abnormality. Counselling is largely by telephone although home visits may be arranged. Support following a subsequent pregnancy is particularly important.

TAMBA (Twins and Multiple Births Association)
Bereavement Support Group
PO Box 30
Little Sutton
South Wirral
L66 1TH
0932 770 382

Aims: to give encouragement and support to parents of twins, triplets or more
        to increase public awareness of the incidence, effects and specific needs
        to promote greater understanding within the statutory, professional and voluntary organisations
        to advance education and encourage research
        to provide information and publications
        to promote and establish a network of local, regional and national support
        to maintain links with other multiple birth organisations worldwide
        to provide and develop resources to achieve these aims.

Index